ILLNESS AND THERAPY

SPIRITUAL-SCIENTIFIC ASPECTS OF HEALING

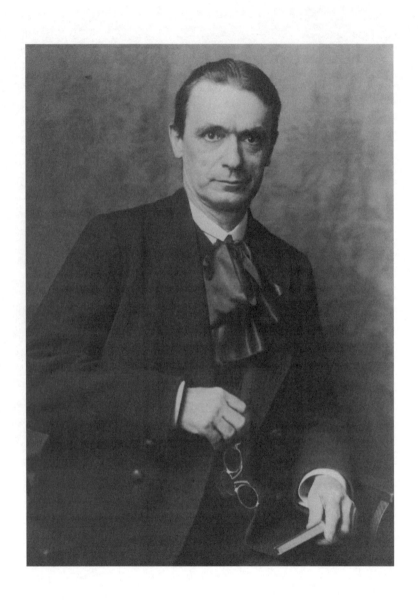

ILLNESS AND THERAPY

SPIRITUAL-SCIENTIFIC ASPECTS OF HEALING

Nine lectures given to physicians and medical students in Dornach between
11 and 18 April 1921 including Rudolf Steiner's notes for the lectures

TRANSLATED BY MATTHEW BARTON

INTRODUCTION BY ANDREW MAENDL, MD, AND
MATTHEW BARTON

RUDOLF STEINER

RUDOLF STEINER PRESS

CW 313

The publishers acknowledge the generous funding of this publication by Dr Eva Frommer MD (1927–2004) and the Anthroposophical Society in Great Britain

Rudolf Steiner Press
Hillside House, The Square
Forest Row, RH18 5ES

www.rudolfsteinerpress.com

Published by Rudolf Steiner Press 2013

Originally published in German under the title *Geisteswissenschaftliche Gesichtspunkte zur Therapie* (volume 313 in the *Rudolf Steiner Gesamtausgabe* or Collected Works) by Rudolf Steiner Verlag, Dornach. Based on shorthand transcripts by Helen Finckh. This authorized translation is based on the 5th German edition of 2001 which was edited by Eva-Gabriele Streit, MD, and Doerte Mehrling

Published by permission of the Rudolf Steiner Nachlassverwaltung, Dornach

A catalogue record for this book is available from the British Library

ISBN 978 1 85584 384 4

Cover by Mary Giddens
Typeset by DP Photosetting, Neath, West Glamorgan
Printed and bound in Great Britain by Gutenberg Press Ltd., Malta

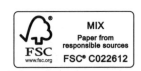

CONTENTS

astrality in respiration, I in warmth. Protein in food and organic protein. Uterus and heart. The relationship between heart activity and fat and carbohydrate metabolism. Tuberculosis. The mercury process. Aspects of medicine production.

LECTURE 7
DORNACH, 17 APRIL 1921

Comprehensive anthroposophic insight into the world as basis for therapeutic assessment. Relationship of the plant to the human organism: using root parts in therapy (gentian, herb bennett, garden lily); herbaceous parts (marjoram); flowers (elder); seeds (caraway). Metamorphosis of the sensory process in metabolism and associated therapeutic perspectives. Principles of metal therapy. Polarity between silver and lead.

LECTURE 8
DORNACH, 18 APRIL 1921

Metal therapy. The concept of poison. Revising the homoeopathic principle. Salt process. Metal process. Radiant actions of the metals. Lead, magnesium, tin, iron, copper, gold, mercury, silver. Answers to questions: treating asthma. Parenteral protein therapy. Colds. Connection between muscles and bones. Enquiries into the sense of taste. Substance and process in the organism. Graves' disease.

LECTURE 9
DORNACH, 18 APRIL 1921

Eurythmy related to the human being configured out of the cosmos as therapeutic element: eurythmy therapy.

EDITOR'S PREFACE

The present volume consists of transcripts of what was known as the second medical course, held for physicians, pharmacists and medical students as continuation of and addition to the first medical course. The wide-ranging stimulus which Rudolf Steiner had offered in the fields of medicine, psychology and general study of the human being, which had informed his work from the beginning, had reached a new, great culmination in the twenty lectures of the first medical course given one year before, and published under the title *Introducing Anthroposophical Medicine* (CW 312). This course had come about at the initiative of a participant who, in responding to Rudolf Steiner's suggestions that an intuitive form of medicine was needed, had asked him to provide the foundations necessary for this. This first course gave a powerful impetus to medical work, and led to the founding of the Clinical-Therapeutic Institute in Stuttgart and Arlesheim. Medicines production also got underway at the International Laboratories (in Arlesheim as part of Futurum AG, and in Stuttgart at Der Kommende Tag AG) from which Weleda eventually developed.

Parallel to this second medical course, *Eurythmy Therapy* (CW 315) was also held each afternoon from 12 to 17 April 1921, and physicians were invited to attend this too. The concluding lecture of 18 April (lecture 9 in the present volume) was intended specifically for physicians as introduction to the field of eurythmy therapy. The eurythmy therapy course came about at the initiative of Elisabeth Baumann-Dollfus and Erna van Deventer-Wolfram to whom, from around 1915, Rudolf Steiner had given many suggestions for the targeted use of eurythmy therapy. In the winter of 1920/21, they asked him to provide a systematic basis in this field. Dr Hendrik van Deventer MD, still a medical student at that time, gave the necessary support for this venture on behalf of the physicians. Thus this new anthroposophic therapy could be inaugurated as an important extension of medical and therapeutic measures.

The chronological table of medical lectures and discussions below offers an overview of Rudolf Steiner's lecturing activities in this field:

[GA = Collected works in German]

Date	Venue	Occasion
21 March–9 April 1920	Dornach	First medical course (*Introducing Anthroposophical Medicine*) GA 312
26 March 1920 7 April 1920	Dornach	Q&A on Psychiatry Hygiene as a social issue (both GA 314, *Physiology and Healing*)
7–9 October 1920	Dornach	Lectures on 'Physiological and therapeutic themes based on spiritual science' (GA 314)
11–18 April 1921	Dornach	Second medical course, GA 313 (*Illness and Therapy*)
12–18 April 1921	Dornach	Eurythmy therapy lectures for physicians and eurythmists, GA 315 (*Eurythmy Therapy*)
26–28 October 1922 28 October 1922	Stuttgart	Anthroposophical Basis for the Practice of Medicine (GA 314) Lecture on eurythmy therapy (GA 314)
31 December 1923/ 1 January/2 January 1924 28 August 1923–29 August 1924	Dornach (various cities)	Discussions with anthroposophical physicians on Therapy (GA 314) *The Healing Process* (GA 319)
2–9 January 1924	Dornach	GA 316 (*Understanding Healing*)
21–25 April 1924 21–23 April 1924	Dornach	Easter course, part of above (GA 316) Discussions with medical practitioners (GA 314)
25 June–7 July 1924	Dornach	GA 317 (*Education for Special Needs*)
8–18 September 1924	Dornach	GA 318 (*Broken Vessels*)

Summary of Medical Courses in English Translation (latest editions shown):

GA/CW 312   *Introducing Anthroposophical Medicine* (SteinerBooks 2010)
313   *Illness and Therapy* (Rudolf Steiner Press 2013)
314   *Physiology and Healing* (Rudolf Steiner Press 2013)

INTRODUCTION

There is a great deal of dissatisfaction in medicine today, and this may partly be due to the prevailing view of the human being as a creature composed more or less entirely of complex biochemistry. Deep down most doctors sense that there is a great deal more to human nature. Steiner has given us a path, albeit a difficult one, for discovering deeper aspects of the human being, upon which a true art of healing can be based. The essence of Steiner's approach is holistic, i.e. not confined to sense-perceptible physical phenomena, but encompassing the whole person. In common parlance, terms like soul and spirit—if used at all—are today regarded as something very vague, at most a kind of 'icing on the cake' of physical reality, and produced by it. Steiner has a radically different, non-materialistic yet extremely precise view of the human entelechy, in which the physical body and its functions are embedded in three other aspects: forces of life and growth (etheric body), powers of sentience and sensibility (astral body) and finally powers of spirit, identity and self-realization (the ego or I).

This may sound schematic, but as Steiner is at pains to point out in this volume—known as 'the second medical course'—the interplay between these different aspects is highly complex. In our attempt to understand health and illness we need to trace this complexity with a precision equal at least to that required for understanding the subtlety of physical processes alone. In fact, as Steiner clearly demonstrates here, we cannot understand physical processes fully without insight into these other, invisible configuring powers that work in them and through them.

Always staying true to such complexity and never simplifying for the sake of easy understanding, Steiner asked a great deal of his original audience of medical professionals. Readers today will find a huge wealth of medical ideas and insights here, but none that can be immediately applied in practice without a great deal of effort and application to make them one's own. Each lecture is likely to need several re-readings, perhaps over years, to accompany our own developing insight as doctors into the causes and remedies of diseases.

The first lecture of this volume offers an introduction to the interplay of supersensible and physical aspects in us. Here Steiner presents a paradigm in which the *four* aspects referred to above—of physical, etheric, astral and I—interrelate in different respective ways with the *threefold* human organism of head, thorax and metabolism (which are also the seat or centre, respectively, of our capacities for thinking, feeling and will). It requires a great mobility and fluidity of thinking to grasp the complex dynamic involved in this four-three relationship, but in doing so we unlock a wonderful diagnostic tool that will stand us in good stead in the appraisal of every patient.

I would like to elaborate this a little further here since it is of such key importance for understanding many other insights of Steiner's. Each of the four aspects, as he describes them, exist in a different configuration within each part of the threefold human organism—acting either as 'primary effect' or 'imprint'. The primary effect can be understood as full physical engagement of respective supersensible forces, while the 'imprint' is a looser or freer reflection of these forces in our organism. In the former, such forces act more within physical functions and processes, whereas in the latter they are released to become available for conscious thinking, feeling and will. Each of these three 'soul forces' as Steiner calls them, in turn have a different quality of relationship with the physical body. We can easily get a sense of such difference by comparing the following three activities: forming a mental image of a candle flame (thinking); going out to dig the garden (will); and listening to beautiful music (feeling). Our experience of will is closer to physical activity while calm, contemplative thinking is furthest removed from it. Feeling, which is centred in and involves the response of our rhythmic system (breathing and circulation), lies roughly midway between the two.

To put this all more precisely—as Steiner does—the I, astral body and etheric body act only in a freer way, as imprint, in the head, while the physical is fully engaged there as primary effect. In the chest region, the astral and I are relatively free as imprint while etheric and physical

are more fully engaged in physical processes. In the system of metabolism and limbs, only the I is relatively free as imprint, and physical,
astral and etheric take primary effect there, in deeper engagement with
the physical body.

Grasping these different relationships and qualities of interplay
requires an artistic as much as a scientific sensibility, and interrelating
them all in a way that serves diagnosis and therapy asks us to be
continually alert, like a conductor to his orchestra, to the potentially
huge range and variation in these interactions, their differing harmonies
and discords in each patient. Steiner in fact says that 'nothing so easily
invokes imaginative pictures as observing pathological conditions in the
human being'; and thus he calls on the faculty of imagination not as it is
commonly regarded today—a close cousin to fantasy—but as a tool of
real perception essential to the physician.

Taking all this a little further, in lecture 3 Steiner focuses on the
thoracic region, reminding us that the life forces of the etheric body
work somatically there, and thus in the same way as they work in the
plant. In a plant, of course, since it has no sentient consciousness, etheric
forces of growth are entirely absorbed in physical processes whereas in us
they are released in the head region to sustain thinking and memory. If
we consider illnesses of the chest region, says Steiner, we have to realize
that the rhythmic qualities of the etheric are intrinsically health-giving
(while all illness originates in the astral) and thus we must seek the
origin of respiratory and circulatory disorders *outside* the rhythmic system itself, either in the neurosensory system, the metabolic system or in
external environmental influences. And likewise a cure must of course
start from diagnosis of the real cause of a disorder, and in the system
where it is rooted. For example, pulmonary tuberculosis can be associated with the inappropriate release of the etheric from its somatic
function in the lung. The 'released' etheric, as we saw, sustains our
capacity to form mental pictures, and there may well be good reason,
therefore, why poets such as Keats, living so vividly in the pictorial
imagination, were more susceptible to this disease. At later stages of the
disease, alveoli and lung tissues harden, and Steiner sees this as the result
of forces of ossification issuing from the head and acting on the lungs.

As Steiner points out, illness often arises where the sequence of reciprocal actions of one supersensible aspect on the other is interrupted. The phenomenon of 'serial permeation' involves the I acting on the astral, which in turn acts on the etheric, and the latter in turn on the physical—rather like a descending chain of command. If the I or astral withdraw from this work under various conditions—such as nervous tension for instance—etheric and physical develop too much vitality and burgeon unhindered. This can produce symptoms such as diarrhoea. Steiner recommends prescribing homoeopathic arsenic in such a case, for this induces the astral to re-permeate the etheric and physical bodies. Arsenic has a hardening action—as we can see in the more or less 'mummified' corpses of people poisoned by this substance, and in homoeopathic potency it draws the astral down into a denser state.

In moving from diagnosis to therapy, an infinitely rewarding insight of Steiner's is our complex connection as microcosm with the macrocosm, and how, in consequence, substances drawn from the natural world can be used to redress imbalances in our organism. As just one example of this relationship, he describes the human being as an 'inverse' plant, whose roots relate to the neurosensory system, its leaves to the respiratory and circulation systems, and its flower and seeds to metabolism. Thus certain parts of a plant are used therapeutically to address the part of the human organism to which they correspond, and Steiner gives many specific examples of such actions which are invariably more complex than any fixed schema would allow. Likewise, in the mineral realm, Steiner explores the medicinal actions of different, potentized metals, as well as of plants watered with metal solutions. Every substance in the cosmos from which we originated has its specific relationship with our own bodily configuration. This view of medicine is not a combative one in which a physician seeks to suppress and vanquish a disorder, but instead one which asks the earth and the cosmos for help in restoring an always fluctuating balance. Such help is not solely in the form of material or medicinal substances but naturally also includes a wide range of approaches including psychological support where appropriate. It can also involve something as gentle and non-invasive as forms of movement which Steiner devised, and to which he gave the name eurythmy. Rendering speech sounds 'visible' in the form of whole body movements, eurythmy draws on the original power of the Word

xvi   *   ILLNESS AND THERAPY

from which the world originated, using the healing effects of vowels and consonants to re-organize and re-attune the human organism.

This course of lectures is far from easy to fathom and requires prolonged, intense study—which will be handsomely repaid in diagnostic and therapeutic insights for those who engage fully with it.

Andrew Maendl, MD, and Matthew Barton, February 2013

LECTURE 1

DORNACH, 11 APRIL 1921

I hope that this supplementary course[1] will really augment and enlarge on last year's course, and by the end will crystallize into a number of therapeutic perspectives. My efforts in this course will focus on examining things that formed the subject of our previous observations—human illness and the search for cures—but now from a different angle. However, since we will be looking at things from a different point of view, we will not only discover different aspects but also broaden the scope of our previous studies. In particular, on this occasion I would like to show what happens in the human organization you are all familiar with as anthroposophists, in terms of physical body, etheric body and so forth, when we fall ill and when we recover. Last time I mostly confined myself to presenting the way our inner nature manifests outwardly. This time, in contrast, I will try to show how the diverse levels of the human being are affected by substances external to us, what the real nature of these substances is which can then be used as medicines, and what can act as a medicine by affecting the human organism in other than merely material ways. Here, however, I will first need to offer a proviso by way of introduction.

On the last occasion, when we discussed the same themes, we also spoke in many respects of substances and physical remedies. Now, though, as we come to consider the higher constituting levels of human nature, the supersensible human bodies, we will need to speak about substances in a different way. While we refer to them in what I would call an abbreviated way, we will nevertheless have to remember a fact

and principle throughout: that we cannot assume the nature of substance to be as the scientific community commonly regards it today if
we really wish to understand our relationship to our environment, and
what characterizes us in a state of health and sickness. Rather than
substances *per se*, we must start from processes: developmental processes
rather than finished products. And whenever we speak of substance we
must really visualize how the external sensory appearance that a substance presents to us is in fact nothing other than a process that has
come to rest.

If we have silica before us, for instance, siliceous earth, we initially
regard it as a substance. But we overlook the key thing if in doing so we
picture it as a particular entity with defined boundaries. We only pin-
point the essential thing about it if we consider what is present as a
single, very extensive process throughout the whole universe. This
process can as it were crystallize and come to rest, can culminate in a
kind of equilibrium and, on coming to rest, manifest as silica. It is vital
to consider the mutual effect between processes within us and those
which unfold outside in the universe, with which we stand in continual
reciprocity both in sickness and health.

To establish the basis for embarking on our actual studies tomorrow,
I wish to present today something that can really lead us to ideas about
this reciprocal effect. Here we have to try to understand the nature of
the human being in terms of anthroposophic spiritual science. I will first
express myself somewhat schematically, focusing on what I have often
presented as the threefold human being, but now in really concentrated
localized form in us. We know that the neurosensory system is largely
concentrated in the head, although what is concentrated in the head is
actually also spread out everywhere in us, is present everywhere in us;
that in the head we are mostly, as it were, a being of nerves and senses
but on the other hand that we are also all head, though less so in the
other two realms than in the head. Thus we can picture what we call our
neurosensory system as being localized in the head. But to make good
use, for our present purposes, of the way we understand this human
organization, we should really see the rhythmic system, comprising
everything relating to respiration and circulation, as being in turn
divided into two parts: one part tending more towards the respiratory

system and the other more towards the circulatory system. And then, integrated into this circulatory system, is everything that embodies the connection between our limb system and metabolic system.

If we study the human head we are also in a sense studying the part of the human organism that is mostly our neurosensory aspect. The organization of the human head is very different from that of the other two systems, also in relation to the form of the higher aspects of human nature. If we consider the human head from an anthroposophic perspective, it is a kind of replica or one might even say a deposit of the I, the astral body and the etheric body. And then let us see how the physical body relates to the head. This physical body is in fact, one can say, present in the head in a different way from the physical that is a replica or imprint of the I, the astral body and the etheric body. Here I would like to accentuate the higher nature of these things by drawing attention to the fact that the human head, in its first foundations in the human embryo, is not configured solely by the forces of the parental organism but that cosmic forces are at work in it; that cosmic forces simply work into the human being. A great deal of the parental organism is at work in what we call the etheric forces, yet even there in the etheric, cosmic forces are at work from the pre-birth realm—or we could say from soul-spiritual life prior to conception. And even in the astral and the I there is an after-effect of what lived in the world of spirit before conception. It continues to work by exerting a formative effect on the human head. The I creates its imprint in the human head, the astral body creates its physical imprint, the etheric body likewise creates its physical imprint. Only the physical body, which is of course first acquired only here on the physical earth, is what we can call a prime mover—not an imprint or replica but something of primary effect. If I draw this schematically [Plate 1 top centre] I can say that the human head is formed as an imprint of the I. Within, this organizes itself in a certain way—and we will come back to this organization repeatedly. It initially does so chiefly by inwardly differentiating the head's temperature. In addition, the astral body differentiates itself inside here and is primarily encompassed as organizing force in the gaseous, air-related processes that permeate the head (Fig. 1). Then the etheric body imprints itself; and then what is physical body for the head is a physical

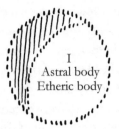

Fig. 1

process, a really physical process (Fig 1, shaded portion). I will indicate this by schematic representation in the drawing of the part of the head that is the bony occiput, with eye level about here.

But again, the physical forces concentrated here extend over the whole head. Here, in this physical part of the human head, we have a real primary physical process. This is not the manifestation of something else but accomplishes its own process. Yet in this physical head process, nevertheless, we have a duality, an interplay of two processes. What happens here is an interplay of two processes that we can only understand if, in our spiritual research, we relate them to certain other processes occurring outside in the universe.

If you take a look at the primary geological process expressed in schist formation—in fact in everything that leads from siliceous earth to schist or shale formation—then you will find, in the forces at work in this process of schist formation originating in silica, the polar opposite process to that which unfolds, on the one hand, in the physical formation of the head. Here you find an important connection between us and our surroundings. Within the human head a process is at work that unfolds in our external surroundings in mineralization. Today, in geology, people have almost—though not quite—come to realize that everything connected with the process of schist formation, of mineralization involving silica, is related to what one might call 'devegetabilization'. We should regard schist formation as a mineralized plant realm. In trying to understand this devegetabilization—which is the same as the earth's schist-forming processes—we grasp the same process that unfolds in a different way here in the human head, in its polar opposite form. There is however an interplay here with another process; and this other process that plays in here has again to be sought in the external world. We have to look for it in limestone formations. Once again, geology, as external science, is now close to accepting the truth that limestone formations are based on a geological process which we could call a 'de-animalization' process, one which is the reversal of what gives rise to the animal. And once again it is the polar opposite process that is at work here. So if we ascribe to silica and calcium—processes that have come to rest in substance—a part in the formation of the physical human head, we have to realize that something plays into this physical head formation that has a very important role in the whole of surrounding nature. At the same time, by way of preparation, we can orient ourselves by seeing silica, on the one hand—and I am speaking of silica as a process that has come to rest—in its key relationship with what happens in the human head; and by seeing limestone formation, on the other hand, or the calcium process that has come to rest, as connected with all that is embodied in the opposite pole and works in polar reciprocity with the other force in the physical human head. These processes, which today we can still find everywhere around us, are connected in the human head with others that we do not find on the earth, and that are present only as imprint in so far as the head is an impression of etheric body, astral body and I.

In relation to these higher members of the human being, we have processes that have come to rest but are not directly earthly processes. The only true earthly process is what I have spoken of here in regard to the physical head *per se*. The other processes are not true earth processes although, as we will see, they are connected to earth processes.

To gain an overview I will now pass straight on to the second realm of the human organism—which we locate in very general terms as the chest. This is the part of the human organism that chiefly encompasses the rhythmic system. Let us immediately divide this schematically firstly into all that comprises the breathing rhythm, and secondly into all that comprises the circulatory rhythm. If we wish to consider as a whole this second part of the human being, we must say the following: all that I have here called the organization of the breathing rhythm in the broadest sense (Fig. 2) is initially an imprint of the I and astral body. [See also Plate 1]

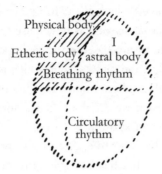

Fig. 2

Just as the head is an imprint of the I, astral body and etheric body, so this breathing rhythm is an impression of the I and astral body, while both physical body and etheric body work together in what takes primary effect here (see shaded part of drawing). The physical body alone has a primary effect in the human head, where the etheric body is also an imprint. In the breathing rhythm system, however, a primary interaction of physical and etheric body is at work, while I and astral body only imprint themselves upon it. This is also largely the case in the circulatory rhythm organization, but in a weaker form, as the whole metabolic organism intrudes into the circulatory system. But here there is already a beginning of what then holds good for the metabolic and limb system. We then have a state of affairs in which the limbs, with all that works into them as metabolism—with the exception of circulation as such, thus of the movement present there—are fundamentally an imprint of the I and an interplay of physical body, etheric body and astral body (Fig. 3). Thus we can say that in considering the human chest system the imprint organization present there is really only what relates to I and astral body, while active within it is a primary organization that is not merely physical now, but shows the physical to be informed and structured by the etheric. This is more strongly so in the breathing rhythm while in the circulatory rhythm we have something else working in from the metabolic system. [See also Plate 1]

You can see this at work in various types of interplay in the different parts of the human being. In these different physical realms, which we call the head system, chest system and limb system, we find different modes of interaction between the levels or bodies which in spiritual

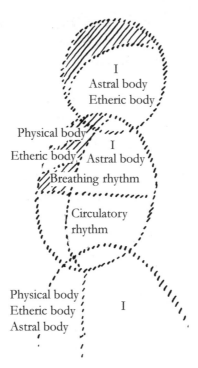

Fig. 3

science we call the physical body, etheric body, astral body and I. The human head, as process, is really largely physical body, while all that is not physical body works as an imprint of the I, astral body and etheric body. Our middle system is largely an interplay of physical body and etheric body, and what is not either physical or etheric body there is an imprint of the I and astral body. The metabolic and limb system is really entirely an interplay of physical body, etheric body and astral body, and an imprint of the I, but, as I have said, works also into the other systems, in interaction with them (see Fig. 3).

Now we must firstly consider how the middle system is informed by the process we illustrated in relation to the physical, the physical head organization, as participation of the silica process that has come to rest. Here we find the remarkable fact that in the middle system the process of silica formation has a stronger, more widespread effect. In the head its action is finer, subtler. Here in the middle system it works in a stronger, more widespread and in a sense more differentiated way. And it works most strongly of all in the metabolic and limb system. So if we now consider the process we have seen as being related to silica, we find that it works most strongly where it is required to aid the I—we will see the reciprocal effect with other processes too—in regard to the action of the autonomous I that has only its imprint in our physical metabolic system. This silica-engendering process works most strongly where it is required to aid the I, in the action of this I upon the metabolic and limb system. Thus this process, which can be characterized in terms of silica, works somewhat more weakly where it only needs to aid the astral body, and most weakly of all where it need only help the etheric body—that is, in the head.

One might put this the other way round, too: in relation to the process we must regard as coming to rest in silica, we find that its action is most material in the head organization, while it works there most weakly in relation to its dynamic impetus or force. But where it works most weakly as force, it takes strongest effect in approaching a static state within substance. Thus if we see silica as the substance present there, we must say that its effect is strongest in the head. If, in contrast, we see it as the outward sign of a process, we have to say that its weakest influence is in the head. Where the strongest material effect exists, the weakest dynamic influence occurs. In our middle system, material and dynamic effect are roughly in equilibrium. And in relation to the metabolic and limb system, the dynamic effect largely has the upper hand: here we have the weakest material effect and the strongest dynamic influence; and thus the process which gives rise to silica really permeates the whole human being with an organizing effect. Having asked about the nature of the reciprocal relationship between the physical head organization and our external surroundings, we can then go on to enquire into the nature of the reciprocal interplay between our middle system—in so far as it is organized as breathing rhythm—and the world around us.

If we wish to study and understand the human head, we have to look at the two processes in earth formation whereby limestone and silica— or if you like silicic acid—arise. We will be looking at this in closer detail. The aspect of us that is less external, less peripheral, and lies more internally, the rhythmic organization of the breathing system, is, as we saw, a primary interplay of physical and etheric into which the I and astral are woven as impressions. Nowhere in our external surroundings, initially, do we find anything that directly embodies this as a natural process. Or at least this is not usually so. If we wish to find a process characteristic of what occurs there through this unique interplay of I, astral body—which are more or less free through their imprinting action—and what acts in a primary way there as an interaction of physical and etheric, this whole interplay can only be properly sought in the external world if we ourselves first engender it. When we burn plant substances and thereby obtain plant ash, the fire and ash-forming process, the process reflected and embodied in such burning and engendering of ash, and in the coming to rest of the ash—we will speak in a moment of different kinds of ash—is related to the breathing process in a way similar to that in which the silica process is related to the process occurring physically in the head. And if we wish to render the correlation to this ash-forming process effective in the rhythmic breathing process, we naturally cannot introduce it into the breath—we can never do this in the human organism—but must instead introduce it into what is, as it were, its other pole. If I draw this [see Plate 1, right] then we have here the rhythmic breathing process and rhythmic circulation process. In the rhythmic breathing process, plant ashes characterize the active processes. But we have to activate these plant ash processes on a roundabout route via the metabolism at the other pole, in the rhythmic circulatory organism (see Fig. 4). We have to incorporate these plant ashes—in other words their dynamic forces—into the circulatory rhythm so that they can then call forth their polar counter-image in the rhythmic breathing process.

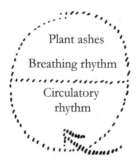

Fig. 4

These relationships reveal themselves to direct perception as being of eminent importance for understanding the human organism. Just as we saw that what is present in the silica-forming process is closely connected with the whole human being, by applying this now to the plant ash-forming process we gain a picture of this middle system in us, which, in turn, is in a sense dual in nature, having both a breathing and a circulatory rhythm.

We gain an idea of this if we say that in the upper rhythm, that of breathing, the structure of the organs concerned is largely determined by a process that is polar opposite to the one revealed when we burn plant material and thereby obtain ash. In the rhythmic breathing process there is, one can say, a continual battle going on against the forming of plant ash, but a battle that does not occur without penetration of the organism by the opposite of this process, in a way that really challenges it. As human beings we live upon an earth in which there are these silica and calcareous processes. If these processes were to fill us we would not be human beings. We are human beings by virtue of bearing within us processes that are polar opposite to these—in other words we can counter the silica formation process and bear its opposite pole within us, and likewise counter the calcium-forming process by bearing its opposite pole within us. We bear these poles within us by virtue of our head formation, which works through the whole human being in different degrees as I described. Through our breathing rhythm we combat the plant ash-forming process. We carry within us the opposite of this plant ash-forming process. When we consider these things it will scarcely be surprising that, to put it somewhat crassly, each impetus invokes a counter-impetus. It is quite clear therefore that if I intensify the silica-forming process in the organism, the counter-effect will be modified accordingly; and it is equally clear that if I introduce the product of the combustion process into the organism, a corresponding counter-effect will be created. This leads to the big question as to how we can gain control over this action and counteraction. In abstract terms, this is something I always express by saying that we first have to recognize what processes are actually at work in the human organism—extending as far as the I—and what processes are at work outside us, outside the human organism. These processes are differentiated inside and outside us. But inside and outside they are polar opposite to each other. The moment something which, by its intrinsic nature should lie outside of my skin is inside my skin, or the moment something works from outside inwards—even if this is just a slight pressure on the body—that by rights should not do so, this elicits an inner counteraction. And at that moment it is my task to create an inner counteraction of this kind to whatever has entered from without. If for instance I find that instead of the normal silica-countering process this process has become excessive or too intense, I need to regulate it from without by administering the relevant substance and invoking the counter-response—which then arises by itself.

These things gradually lead us to insight into the reciprocal relationship between us and our natural surroundings. If you can really grasp how the dynamic involved in the silica-forming process reciprocates and responds to the I when the latter seeks to act through the limbs and metabolism, and if moreover you know that the material effect in the silica-forming process works most strongly in the head, at the same time seeing that its dynamic action is only needed to a lesser degree to aid the I in the human head, then you will be able to gain insight into how this I works in different degrees within us.

If we now consider the relationship of the human I to the metabolic and limb system, we find there, really, the source of human egotism. This system of human egotism also of course includes the sexual system. And the I acts to penetrate the human entity with egotism precisely also on the roundabout route through the sexual system.

If you grasp this you will say that there is a certain opposition between the way in which the I uses silica in order to act upon us from the limb system, and the way in which this same I works from the human head through silica—where, in a sense, it acts without egotism. If we study this through spiritual science, we see a differentiating effect here.

If I depict this remarkable effect schematically, I must say that what the I does in us when acting through silica from the limb system (Fig. 5, red)—now as a real organizing element—is fundamentally a cohesive effect on us, as it were binding all fluids present in us into an undifferentiated unity, and giving rise to an undifferentiated, unified whole. [See also Plate 1]

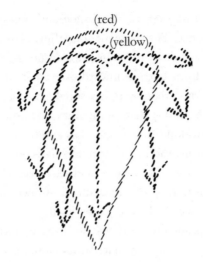

Fig. 5

Everything that, while involving the same process, forms silica in the least intensive way in terms of dynamic force, acts in the opposite way (see Fig. 5, yellow), exerting a differentiating and radiating action. From below upwards the human being is encompassed, unified and rendered undifferentiated through silica, while from above downwards he is differentiated into separate aspects. This means however that the action of forces organically present in the head is differentiated for the different organs. These forces are in a sense stimulated by the silica process intrinsic to the head to work as they should, to distribute themselves appropriately to heart, liver and so forth.

Here we meet a process which, in working from below upwards, merges and jumbles everything up in us and, when it works from above downwards, structurally separates everything, as it were ruling the organism and organizing each separate organ appropriately. If we then perceive what occurs in us through this jumbling up on the one hand and, on the other, this driving apart into the diverse organs—that is, a differentiating mode of organization in contrast to a synthesizing one— and see how this can be irregular in each individual, then we gradually learn to treat a patient with this in mind when a disorder arises. We will see this in more detail in the lectures that follow. But in examinations of this kind we must really be extremely careful. For what does an external scientific approach actually discover in examining the human organism?

Scientists state, for example, that there is silica in the human organism, fluorine, magnesium and calcium. External scientific analysis shows that we have silica in our hair, blood and urine. Now let us first take these two: silica is present in our hair and urine.

An external approach considers that there is nothing else to be said except that we find silica in human hair, and then again silica in human urine. But the fact that some substance or other is present somewhere is not the important thing. The silica in our hair is there as a source of activity. We do not have hair for no reason, but from our hair forces pass in turn to the organism—and in fact the very finest, subtlest forces pass from our hair back into the organism. We have silica in our urine as something that is otherwise superfluous: what is not used is excreted there. In fact, silica in urine is a matter of indifference. It is not active there but is just in the process of being expelled as something that should not be active, of which there is too much. The urine contains silica that should not be in the organism and which therefore has not the slightest significance for it. It is the same when we examine any distinct substance, let us say magnesium. If there were no magnesium in our teeth, they would not be teeth at all. In the magnesium process live forces that are most closely involved in building up the teeth. You heard this in Professor Roemer's talk.[2] But according to materialistic science, magnesium is also in milk. Yet there it has no significance. By its very nature milk is strong enough to expel the magnesium it contains. Magnesium as such has no intrinsic place in milk. We can analyse it, of course, but in fact the milk-producing process can arise through the fact that it can expel magnesium forces. We only learn something about this remarkable contrast between the processes of dental development and milk production by knowing that magnesium belongs intrinsically and dynamically to the dental development process. In the milk-producing process, on the other hand, it is surplus to requirements and is expelled. Things are similar with fluorine, for example, which plays a key part in dental enamel, and which is essential to our understanding of the process of dental evolution. It is also present in the urine, but there as excretion process, and without significance to this. The fluorine present in the urine is in fact what the organism is powerful enough to excrete because it cannot use it.

A merely physical analysis of whether a particular substance is present somewhere really doesn't tell us anything of importance. We always need to know whether something is playing an active part at the right place or whether it is just present because it has been expelled or excreted. That is the decisive thing. The key thing is that we acquire such concepts so as to understand health and sickness in the human being and other organic entities. Yet speaking in a more accessible way always requires us to dispense with these aids, because in our age people in general have not been educated to grasp subtler concepts. It becomes necessary to speak more abstractly, and therefore less comprehensibly. We frequently become incomprehensible when combating materialism. But if we descend—we might still descend into quite different regions as well—into the characteristic nature of realms which scientists really ought to know, whose facts are available to them and can be studied and analysed, then precisely through spiritual science we can demonstrate that the idea of particular substances which chemical and physical analysis locates in particular places in fact leads to nothing but error.

This was by way of introduction. We will speak further of these things tomorrow.

LECTURE 2

As I said yesterday, we will consider the human being in relation to his supersensible nature, on this occasion focusing on phenomena of pathology and therapy from this perspective. Yesterday we characterized the physical body by stating that physical activity is only really present in our head. If we wish to properly understand this physical body we must naturally also rise one level higher to consider the etheric body in a fully specific way. Insight into the human being shows us that a distinct and separate action of the physical body exists only in the head. In the other bodies or aspects of the human organism the physical body works in more undifferentiated interplay with the higher, supersensible bodies. In the head, therefore, the supersensible levels as such can function in or through thinking, feeling and will because they are first imprinted in the head—thus have their etheric, astral and also I imprint there. These are present—as imprints, or if you like as pictures of the supersensible aspects. Only the physical body as yet makes no imprint or replica of itself, doing so only during the course of life. This is why we can say that the physical body acts in the head in a purely physical way, while in the other human limbs no purely physical action as such exists.

Several people did not understand yesterday when I said that the I makes an imprint of itself. The I makes an imprint for itself—this is something we will properly understand only as long as we do not interpret it in the ordinary sense, in other words too physically. What the I creates for itself as imprint while remaining free, as it alone does in the limb and metabolism system, is not something we can examine by comparing it for instance with a plaster cast. No, the imprint which the I creates is a very fluid one. In fact you'll get a better idea of it when you're moving than when you stand still. The imprint created by the I is one acting within a system of forces that arises as we move within a whole context of forces—also when we hold ourselves upright. Here lies the physical imprint of the I. So you should not seek this imprint of the I in anything comparable to a plaster cast. It is, rather, an imprint in a system of forces. And this, ultimately, is what it also is in the head, though here in a different system of forces. Yesterday, in fact, I pointed out that the I imprints itself into the head's temperature conditions—thus in the way the head's various organs are permeated by different temperatures. That is the I imprint. This I imprint is also an imprint within a system of forces, but here a system of temperatures. Thus the I creates imprints for itself in the most diverse ways. Where it remains free of other contributory effects in the human organism, it makes a pure, or you could say a mechanical, imprint of forces. The I creates for itself an imprint of balancing and dynamic forces in relation to our limb and metabolic system. But here we must also consider that we are actually different in nature depending on whether we stand still, walk or even swim. Unfortunately people take far too little account of this. In fact we must say of many things not sufficiently considered from a spiritual-scientific perspective that they clearly show us the self-imposed limits of modern science, the real facts researchers fail to engage with. In this regard, for instance, I was interested in something which I will only mention now in passing—and will leave as a question to be answered during these lectures. I studied the customary literature and found it stated everywhere, somewhat disarmingly, that there is little difference between the volume of nitrogen in inhaled or exhaled air. This is stated more or less everywhere. But it is not true. The recorded volumes testify immediately to the untruth of the statement, showing that more nitrogen is exhaled than inhaled. But because materialism has no idea what to make of this difference, it cancels it out with a shrug of dismissal. Such things happen in modern research. As I said, I will just leave this here as a question, and return to it later.

Now, however, I would like to look at the human etheric body. It is self-evident that a merely physical scientific approach cannot arrive at a differentiated consideration of this etheric body. But if you can assure yourself of the existence of this etheric body, you will have to admit that it would be an odd thing to see the physical body as one blurred mass without differentiating between, say, the stomach, heart and liver. But that is what we do in relation to the etheric body if we posit it as a general and scarcely differentiated entity, a sort of mist. We must study it properly, and today we will see how study of it is connected with an essential idea—which we considered from a different angle during our last medical course. This idea is one I would like to touch on today from a more spiritual-scientific perspective.

If we consider the ether in general, of which the human etheric body is naturally a part—a distinct configuration of it—we find, as you already know from the general literature of spiritual science, that it is not undifferentiated but initially comes to our attention in the form of four ether types: warmth ether, light ether, chemical ether and life ether. Light ether is a word coined, of course, from the point of view of people who can see. The primary and most striking effect of this ether is connected with light for those who have the sense of sight. In fact it contains other effects we overlook only because most of us can see. If most of humanity were blind, we would have to give another name to this ether since its other aspects would come to the fore instead; and for blind people this is actually the case.

The third type of ether is the chemical ether. This acts primarily in the so-called 'chemical' part of the spectrum. When we speak of the chemical ether we should not think only of, say, forces active in processes of chemical synthesis but also of forces that are polar opposite to these. Ether forces are always polar opposite to those acting in physical substances. Thus, whenever a chemical synthesis arises, the etheric forces act in an analytic way. This means that analytic forces are present everywhere in synthesizing forces. In undertaking a chemical analysis, the spiritual researcher will always find the following. We do a chemical analysis—I'll draw this schematically—and chemically isolate the constituents of a substance: [See also Plate 2]

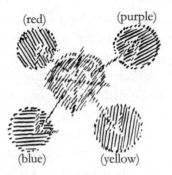

(red) (purple)

(blue) (yellow)

Fig. 6

And then the ether body remains afterwards—in a manner all the more compact due to synthesis of the ether forces—in exactly the same way as the soul and spirit remain after we die. Anyone who undertakes a chemical analysis with what I will call eyes of spirit sees after he has isolated the constituents of a chemical substance the remaining ghost of this substance in a proportionally more condensed and compacted form. I only say this to show you that chemical ether forces should not be regarded merely as chemical forces, as synthesizing and analysing forces, but always as their polar opposite aspect. And then, as another distinct type of ether, we have the life ether, which is the actual animating element in all organic life.

> Life ether
> Chemical ether
> _____
> Light ether
> Warmth ether

Now this ether is an entity generally present in the universe, and as such cannot of course be perceived by directly physical means. In this respect, scientists have grown a little more candid than they used to be, acknowledging that theories about the ether cannot be posited on merely physical modes of observation. Countless such theories were proposed in the past, but proponents of relativity now state that there is no such thing as ether—the world must be explained without it. In other words, they have become more honest, agreeing with Einstein[3] that physical observations do not lead us to ether, but nor do they lead us to any other mode of observation. Since people have ceased to have any perception of the ether, they now simply exclude it from consideration.

What in fact happens is this: once a supersensible element has created an imprint in the physical and sensory realm, then this imprint becomes permeable for the corresponding supersensible activity. You see, therefore, that the general ether creates for itself an imprint in the aqueous realm of the human head. What we must regard as the brain's aqueous content should not be thought of as merely undifferentiated fluid, but is just as thoroughly organized as our solid limbs. It is really a very odd way to view the human being if we see him more or less in the same terms as drawings depict him. If we map the human body, with liver and stomach, such a drawing is really only a silhouette of something that is in fact intrinsically interwoven with aqueous and gaseous parts. What we draw is really only a depiction of, as it were, small grains embedded in a greater flux. It does not even compose ten per cent of us. In reality of course, in physical terms, we are just as much water, air and warmth organisms. And within us the water or fluid is just as fully organized as the solid parts. We never draw this in anatomical or physiological drawings. The substance composing our aqueous content is of course involved in a continual process of dissolution and renewal. The form of it is, you can say, only configured for a moment, but it is still structured. This aqueous part of the human head is indeed where we find the imprint of the etheric. To draw a diagram I would therefore have to draw the physical activity, which is most strongly developed in the occiput, more or less like this (see Fig. 7, shaded); it radiates through the whole organism, of course. [See also Plate 2]

Naturally it penetrates the whole organism. Then, for the aqueous part I would have to draw the rest like this (Fig. 7, yellow). It is organized, thoroughly permeated, so that this aqueous element is an imprint of something etheric in nature. Whatever is an imprint becomes permeable in this way. Since the intrinsic nature of the eye is created by light, as Goethe describes so clearly,[4] it is permeable to light. This is not merely a metaphor but profound wisdom: the eye did indeed arise from light. We can even trace this in embryology, seeing that the eye develops and is organized from outside inwards. Because it is organized and structured by light, it is permeable to light. But over and above

(light shading)   (red)

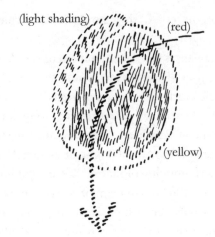

(yellow)

Fig. 7

this, the head's aqueous organization means that it is permeable to the etheric because it is an imprint arising from the ether. And so we can say that the etheric is able to pass through the head here (see Fig. 7, above, red arrow) without in any way being obstructed or disturbed in its passage, and can penetrate into the rest of the human organism.

This is something we can certainly observe through spiritual science. But we also need to consider how this law is modified. This part of the human head is in fact only permeable for the warmth ether and light ether. Only the warmth ether and light ether can work upon the human head from without. The warmth ether does not act directly via heat radiation but affects the human head through the fact that we are embedded in a particular climatic region. In other words, instead of seeking the action of the warmth ether on the human head in relation to whether you are perspiring or not, you must ascertain whether you live in an equatorial, temperate or cold zone of the earth. You see, the warmth ether's connection with the human head goes far deeper than merely streaming in from without. As far as physiology is concerned—psychology involves other aspects that go beyond our present scope—we must think in similar terms of the influence of the light ether on the human organism: this is far more enduring than simple, external light influences. The activity of this light ether passes through the etheric imprint in the human head and exerts an organizing influence throughout the human being. So as we saw, the human head organization is permeable to warmth ether and light ether. It is not quite accurate but nevertheless approximately correct to say that the human head is *somewhat* permeable to chemical ether and life ether. We can neglect this here however, since the outcome is still as I will now describe. The chemical ether and life ether that are present are repulsed by the organization of the head, as you can see from the above. They are repulsed. But instead they pass through the human organism. By virtue of the fact that we live on earth as human beings, we are inwardly filled with life ether and chemical ether.

We can put it like this. The influence of the warmth and light ether streams in from all sides (Fig. 8, descending arrows). The action of the chemical and life ether streams up through the system of metabolism and limbs towards the in-streaming warmth and light ether (Fig. 8, ascending arrows). [See also Plate 2]

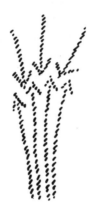

Fig. 8

Just as the organization of the human head is, one can say, somewhat anxiously predisposed to allow in only traces, if possible, of life ether and chemical ether, the metabolic and limb system by contrast really sucks up the life ether and chemical ether from the element of earth. These two types of ether meet within us; and the human organization is such that it culminates in maintaining an ordered separation of these two types of ether: life ether and chemical ether on the one hand, streaming upwards from below, and warmth ether and light ether on the other, streaming downwards from above.

Intrinsic to the human organism is the fact that its lower system in a sense does not organically incorporate what streams in from above—the light ether and warmth ether—except in so far as it streams in by this path. And, equally, nothing may stream in from below to influence something different in nature. Thus, light ether and warmth ether must stream in from outside, life ether and chemical ether must stream in from below, and the organism, sustained as it must be if we are to live within our normal organization, causes an interplay of these two streams. We can begin to understand the nature of this interplay if, firstly, we study people who are distinctly malnourished. Here we gain an impression that resides entirely in the realm of imaginative perception—to which we can easily raise ourselves, however, if the reality of imagination has once been brought home to us in even the subtlest way. In fact nothing so easily invokes imaginative pictures as observing pathological conditions in the human being. Now if we see a malnourished person before us, we find that his metabolic organization—in other words what occurs in the metabolism—binds the ether and does not let it go. If you look, say, at the stomach or liver of a malnourished person, you will find that he retains the life ether and the chemical ether. He binds these ethers to himself, does not let them go, giving rise therefore to a deficiency of upstreaming life ether and chemical ether. In consequence, the light ether and warmth ether press down upon such a person from above, so that his whole organism assumes a condition which previously only existed in the head due to the action of light and warmth ether. These ethers reconfigure the whole organism so that, in a certain sense, it comes to resemble the head organization too strongly. Then a person becomes almost entirely head through malnutrition. He is as it were transformed into being entirely head, and this is of very great importance in the study of malnutrition.

Then, by contrast, we can observe someone suffering from the opposite of malnutrition. These things become apparent in extreme states, and we have to be able to observe them properly. You will no doubt ask what the opposite of malnutrition is. One instance of a condition in which the spiritual researcher finds the opposite of malnutrition is commonly called 'softening of the brain'. Just as malnutrition is due to a person being permeated by what ought to remain in the head, and should only make its way into the upper organism, so in softening of the brain the head is permeated by what should remain in the stomach, does not belong in the brain but in the stomach, and only exerts a duly organizing action in the latter. In other words, the organism is too active in working upon what it assimilates in the process of digestion. It acts on it and converts it excessively, does not sufficiently hold it back before it passes the gateway through which it enters the head. The consequence of this, of course, is that due to too much being as it were poured into the head, more is also eaten than is appropriate for the particular human organization. We can also clearly observe the further effects of such things. Indeed, to gain any insights in the areas we are discussing, it is of very great significance to form an idea of how these processes continue and develop. What happens when these processes, which are really quite normal at the outset—such as eating, digesting, assimilation in the abdomen, transfer towards the head and so forth—continue and exceed the goal normally assigned them by the organism? In a malnourished person, through the irregularity that arises in the lower system, the two ether types work together abnormally, and do so also in an overnourished person through irregularities in the upper system. The two types of ether do not work together as they ought to in the human organism. Due to this inappropriate interplay of the ether working in from outside and the ether rising up from within us, the following occurs: an ether that acts upon us from without but does not cease its action at the right place, instead permeating us more strongly than it should, is toxic for the human organism. It has a poisonous effect on our organization due to the fact that it does not come to a halt at the right place, failing to engage in the right way with the ether rising up from within us.

And likewise, if we study the inner ether, the other type of ether that works from within, this ether has a generally softening effect when it exceeds its due scope. Whereas the toxic effect first mentioned leads to us becoming etherically rigidified, the opposite effect means that we flow out too much, dissolve. Too much life is poured out over us, along with too much of a polar chemical nature. We can no longer preserve ourselves, but soften and dissolve. So here we have two polar effects: the toxic and the softening, dissolving effect. Studying the human being in this way, and asking what he really is, we find that, as far as his physical nature is concerned, he is an organic being that holds asunder the two types of ether in the right way, and also in turn allows them to work together in the right way. The whole human organization is really predisposed to allow the two ether types to work together correctly.

And now we are coming closer to what I meant by saying that we are entirely organized throughout. It is self-evident that we are inwardly differentiated—that is, organized—in relation to water, air and temperature. But we are also differentiated in relation to the ether. In this case, though, the differentiation is a fluctuating one: a continual process and interplay in us of light and warmth ether on the one hand, descending from above downwards, as peripheral impetus, and of life and chemical ether on the other, which pushes up from below as outwards-directed, centrifugal dynamic. This gives rise to the etheric configuration we call the human being—really as a reconfiguration of the vortex, formed as the two types of ether encounter each other. The form you encounter here has to be understood in terms of the interplay of the two types of ether. It is of some importance to [form ideas about human health and sickness] by drawing, specifically, on still less obvious processes such as those of malnutrition and obesity. Clinical obesity does not merely mean that we stuff ourselves. If we have acquired a better than average digestion we are likely to be far less obese than if we have in some way impaired our digestion, so that food is not properly assimilated. As our point of departure, therefore, we can try to focus on what we find by observing these initial processes, which are still very much within normal bounds. At the same time it is also important to say that if we could not fall ill we could not be human beings at all. Illness is simply a continuation or progression beyond due bounds of processes we need, that are indispensable. Human health, we can say, is the condition in which pathological and curative processes are in appropriate equilibrium. We are not in fact only at risk when pathological processes manifest but also when curative processes overshoot their target. Then too we are vulnerable. When introducing a healing process, therefore, it is important not to proceed too radically, which will mean we overshoot our target, suppressing the illness so that, pushed back to zero point, it rebounds instead in the other direction.

In this context it is very striking to see the kinds of instinctive therapeutic approaches people had in former times. Anyone who has studied these things will, I think, acknowledge that wonderful therapeutic approaches existed in ancient cultures, founded on human instincts. Though these were not consciously understood, they certainly existed; and even where we find them in decadent form today, as in ethnic tribes, such lore is still impressive. Not so long ago, gentlemen who were otherwise very scholarly in their own fields caused a stir through their somewhat dilettante preoccupation with such things. A dispute broke out between scholars in Jena and Berlin relating to *Pithecanthropus erectus*. As we know, Virchov[5] argued with Haeckel[6] that the *Pithecanthropus* discovered by Dubois[7] revealed clear signs of healing, of mended bones, which a modern physician can interpret as evidence of an intentionally induced healing process. This was one of Virchov's main objections, leading him to the hypothesis that this *Pithecanthropus erectus* was cured by a physician; and that physicians must therefore have been around in those times—resembling Virchov himself no doubt—who initiated the cure by externally applied means. He argued, therefore, that *Pithecanthropus* was not some missing link preceding the human being *per se*, but that this was a human being. A proper physician might just feasibly have cured an ape, but this was not accepted. The counter-argument, by the other scholars stomping around in just as dilettante a way—since all they did was express general suppositions—ran as follows. Spontaneous cures also occur in animals, without human intervention, and can easily resemble the cure that occurred in the case of the *Pithecanthropus*.

I cite this example only to show the lack of clarity prevailing today. Much was written and published about this in the early nineties of the last century; and academic disputes of this kind are indicative of the type of arguments we often meet today.

In the instinctive ideas of a more primitive humanity, therefore, we do indeed find what could be called 'instinctive therapy'. From such instinctive therapeutic approaches emerged a very important principle: that the art of healing must not be imparted to anyone unreliable because, at the same time, one would have to reveal the art of making people ill. This principle was rooted in primal medical practices, and was very strictly adhered to. It is also one of the reasons why ancient medical teachings were shrouded in a certain secrecy.

Pathological processes, therefore, are nothing other than a further development of processes indispensable in a healthy person. If we were unable to fall sick then we could not think or feel either. Everything that ultimately comes to expression in the psyche as thinking and feeling is, in clinical terms, a system of forces that becomes pathological when it exceeds its proper bounds. And the other thing to be aware of is that an intrinsically physical process only occurs in one part of the human head. This physical process occurring in the human head is a necessary concomitant to our human I experience. When this process is disturbed, or in other words where a vitalizing process overwhelms this purely physical process in us, the I is in a certain sense dulled and numbed, also in our conscious mind. And all cases where a person becomes delirious, mentally incapacitated, or similar, result partly—and must be correspondingly diagnosed—from something that has occurred as a purely physical process. Of course, other organic causes can also exist.

You see therefore that what is initiated by the human head and from there streams through the whole organism is a purely physical process which, at the moment death occurs, floods the whole organism. This moment is always present in the human head, or at least emanates from it in a centralizing fashion. But it is paralysed by the vitalization process rising from the other part of the organism. We actually continually bear in us the forces that cause death, and we could not be an I without bearing these death forces. We could only desire to be physically immortal, as humans physically existing upon the earth, if we relinquished the capacity for self-awareness. It is necessary, as I have pointed out, to develop certain intimate observational capacities so as to provide external verification of this. At the same time, however, it would be very useful if a great number of doctoral theses studied how rejuvenation treatments, which counter ageing, affect a person's state of mind and soul. I have nothing against rejuvenation cures as such, for some might well find it worthwhile to exchange a few more years of life at an advanced age for a little feeble-mindedness. But anyone who wishes to study the real nature of processes at work in illness and health must consider these things—they do indeed exist but are overlooked in the same way as the fact that we exhale a greater volume of nitrogen than we inhale. The more we engage with these subtleties of the human organization, the more we begin to gain insight into processes of illness that are in fact nothing other than a coarser manifestation of these subtler processes. What I have identified here is just a transposition of these subtler processes into a more starkly apparent form. We have to see that the I counteracts, for as long as possible, what works in us, permeates us, as physical process; and that this I is intrinsically bound up with this reactive function. It opposes this physical process as long as the latter does not become too strong. This physical process is implicit in continual dying within the human organism, and in what ultimately manifests in death. In fact, if the physical process hypertrophies, as it were, so that the I can no longer control it, the I is compelled to leave the physical body—which can of course occur at an earlier stage of life if an excessive physical effect arises somewhere in us, with further ramifications throughout the body. And so we can say that the human I is intimately connected with death: [See Plate 2]

I—death

You can in fact study the I most precisely by studying death—though not in the general and nebulous way people imagine death, which allows you to take all sorts of liberties. The way people picture death today can be likened to how they imagine the destruction of a machine, for it seems to them that death is just cessation. They do not picture the real process involved, and so conceive of death as the destruction of a machine. But this is of no help at all. Instead we must engage with what actually, specifically occurs. Cessation of life is not death, but—as far as the human being is concerned—death is as I have described it here, while for animals it is something quite different. Those who regard death in the human being and animal as something identical are doing the same thing as someone who finds a razor and tries to carve a joint with it, since a blade is a blade. They think that death is death, but in fact it is quite different in us than it is in animals, as I have tried to show. The animal, which has no I at all, but only an astral body, has a quite different kind of death, arising from the very different nature of its astral body.

Illness is a condition in which death-bringing forces are diluted, checked or suppressed in a normal organism. Just as death is connected with the I, so illness goes hand-in-hand with the human being's astral body: [See Plate 2]

Astral body—illness

The astral body is the seat of all that is connected with illness. And what the astral body perpetrates is in turn impressed into the etheric body. This is why illness comes to expression as imprint in the etheric body, although the etheric body itself has no immediate connection with illness.

Earlier I described the irregular and disordered interplay and confluence of the two types of ether. But this irregularity is itself in turn merely the effect of the astral body imprinting itself in the etheric body. If we take a closer look at this we can trace it back to the astral body. Going into this in more detail, we have a polar aspect that counters illness, and this is health: [See Plate 2]

Etheric body—health

It will be better not to define health to begin with, but by analogy you can see something that is increasingly clear in spiritual research: health is assigned to the etheric body in the same way as illness to the astral body. And just as death and the I belong together, so healing or curing means having the capacity to create counteractions in the etheric body to the illness-inducing influences emanating from the astral body. To paralyse the forces of the astral body, with their illness-inducing influences, we have indeed to work from the etheric body.

Then there is a fourth thing, which in a certain sense is polar opposite to death. First, however, I need to point out that human death occurs quite specifically when our whole inner organization has passed over into the physical realm in a way that renders impossible the initiation of any kind of nutritional process, seen in the most radical sense. This is the death that occurs in old age. Death in old age is really the organism's loss of capacity to absorb substances. This phenomenon has not yet really been discerned—and is, or can be, so little observed because people usually die beforehand through other causes than wasting or marasmus in its fullest 'flowering', or more aptly 'unflowering'. But really a failure of nutrition is at work. The body can no longer accomplish nutrition properly since it has become too physical; and thus the polar opposite of death is nutrition, and nutrition in us is assigned to the physical body: [See Plate 2]

Physical body—nutrition

The different levels work back upon each other. Nutrition accomplished in the physical body works back upon the etheric body, and is therefore also connected with a curative effect. This is again something that works back as reaction on what proceeds from the astral body.

If we try to directly observe in daily life what I have now described, we can also verify it from the other perspective. If you take something discovered through our earlier spiritual-scientific enquiries, you will need to make a clear division here: [See Plate 2]

I—death
<u>*Astral body—illness*</u>
Etheric body—health
Physical body—nutrition

For during sleep, at least in relation to the head and respiratory organization, the I and astral body sunder themselves entirely from the physical body. This is not true in relation to the metabolic and circulatory organization, where these aspects remain connected. It is not precisely true to say that the I and astral body depart. Instead—and I touched on this often in the past, many years ago already—it is true to say that, in relation to the head organization, the I and astral body emerge from the physical body and etheric body during sleep, but thereby penetrate the metabolic and circulatory organization all the more. A reconfiguration occurs, as parallel phenomenon to the alternation of day and night on earth. In fact it is true, of course, that the whole earth is not simultaneously plunged into night or day, but that the locus of day and night keeps changing. The same applies to what is really a precise imprinting of day and night upon human sleeping and waking. While we are awake, our physical and etheric bodies in the head and breathing organism are intimately connected with the I and astral body; whereas in sleep the physical and etheric bodies of the metabolic and circulatory organism are far more intimately connected with the I and astral body than is the case while we are awake. A rearrangement occurs, a rhythmical reconfiguration occurring between sleep and waking.

But now, in sleep, we can see—at least for the upper human organization—that the astral body departs with the I. We may sometimes observe that a person's astral body and I seize hold too strongly of his head organization, or perhaps also his respiratory organization. They take too strong a hold, grasp it too strongly, and here the astral body is acting out of its illness-inducing forces. Then we can find it is necessary to take measures to drive this astral body out of the head and respiratory organizations again, to drive it out so that they separate from each other in a certain sense and allow normal conditions to be re-established. As one can observe, intake of very small doses of phosphorus and also sulphur can induce this. Small doses of these substances act to drive out an astral body embedding itself too strongly in the physical and etheric body: the sulphur acts more on the astral body, the phosphorus more on the I—which, because it permeates and organizes the astral body, really works as one with the latter. Here we can directly perceive what is happening in a person with a morbid state whose symptoms we can describe as an excessive tendency to sleep. Thus, if we find a pathology which includes symptoms of comatose conditions, then this is indicative of a need to work, as I said, with phosphorus and sulphur.

If the opposite condition arises, with its seat in the metabolism and circulatory organism, in which the astral body and the I intervene too little in the physical body, so that one wishes to invite these gentlemen to get more involved, to work a little harder and more actively, then we need the action of not too highly diluted arsenic. Here we work to draw in the astral body into the physical organism.

The suggestions I am making are drawn from a detailed, holistic view of the human being. If the astral body becomes too inwardly active, thus working too strongly on the physical body, this can be remedied with sulphur and phosphorus; when, in contrast, the astral body works too weakly, becoming too inwardly lazy so that the etheric body predominates due to its* insufficient power of resistance to what works from below, then one can remedy this with arsenic.

Here, then, we have two polar opposites in the phosphorus-and-sulphur action and that of arsenic. But now we can also find that merely regulating things from one pole or the other will not solve the problem, since an irregularity in one part of the human being immediately causes a counter-effect and is perpetuated in an opposite irregularity somewhere else. The disorder in the upper organization soon expresses itself in a disorder in the lower organization. And this interplay of two disorders is something that—well, forgive me, the expression is not appropriate for life in general but just for a clinical view of things—is really most fascinating: this disordered interplay where the two activities are not in equilibrium but where instead too weak an influence from above calls forth too strong a one below, or vice versa. These things are polar opposite not only as regards their level and direction but also of course their intensity. This interplay is the most complex thing at work in us. If we understand this fully, we therefore find it necessary to re-establish balance by invoking the forces at work in us, rebalancing them again. And this is aided by the action of antimony. The actions of antimony, which today I believe are more or less overlooked in mainstream medicine, and work in a way that people no longer understand—though they were known in former times—are largely due to their capacity to bring their actions to bear within us, creating an equilibrium point of sorts. It really is extremely interesting to observe the opposite mode of action of phosphorus, arsenic and antimony in relation to what occurs in us through them. Whatever comes to a certain state of rest as a substance in the outer world expresses its true nature when its action takes effect within the human being. For only then do we really see what is still alive in it, whereas an external perspective only shows us what has, as it were, coagulated as residue of its developmental process. If you look at arsenic outwardly, it really embodies in the external world the end of a process whose beginning can be found within us. We can never gain full insight into a substance

---

* Translator's note: It is not entirely clear here whether the pronoun refers to the etheric body or, more likely, the astral body.

we observe in the outer world if we do not know, at the same time, how it acts inside the human organism. As well as the field of chemistry there is also one of anti-chemistry. Chemistry only means looking from one angle, from behind, at an entity that has a front and back. A being with a back also has to be observed from the front, and only then, by comparing these two aspects, can we gain an impression of its totality. Having only observed what lives in a substance by examining its rear view, we must then also go round to the front and take a look at how it acts in the human organism. Besides pursuing chemistry we also need anti-chemistry, and in the interplay of both we gain insight into the true underlying realities. We will look at this in more detail tomorrow.

LECTURE 3

DORNACH, 13 APRIL 1921

STUDY of disease ought to focus on the domain that belongs intrinsically to it—disorders that most clearly reveal an inappropriate influence of what we call the astral body. The disorders I am thinking of, where such influences of the astral body are most apparent, are those we locate within the area enclosed by the chest or ribcage. This domain is simultaneously the most important for the study of illness yet also the most problematic for healing or for understanding how healing occurs. This is the region of the human being which in recent times has most clearly revealed shortcomings in medical practice such as those Dr Scheidegger[8] highlighted in the lecture he was kind enough to give to the assembled physicians during our first medical course. He showed the extent to which modern developments in medicine have led to advances in the field of pathology, yet at the same time to a certain nihilism in the therapeutic field. In fact, his significant comments require us to give particular attention to the aspects we will consider today.

Disorders of the human chest and circulatory region are, in certain respects, very different both from disorders of the head organs, the human neurosensory system, and from true metabolic disorders. Nevertheless they are intimately related to both of these. The head organization requires special treatment because, as we have seen, it is permeable to our etheric, astral and I nature. The organs of the chest are no longer permeable to the etheric, but only to our astral and I nature. There, in the organs of the thorax, physical body and etheric body work intimately together, and this collaboration is a unified whole. In the human chest organism we no longer find a sum of intrinsically physical processes at work, but rather an interaction of etheric and physical. What occurs there, and is of particular importance to consider for the chest, is basically a kind of plant development. This plant growth, though, is very much hidden within or modified by everything else related to it in the human organism. Nevertheless, we must take particular account of this plant process, which in turn encounters everything proceeding from the human astral body and I, and works in reciprocal interaction with them.

Yesterday I said that the astral body is the primary carrier of the morbid principle in us, and therefore the human chest region continually gives rise to the influx and influence of what actually causes disease. Within the organs of the thorax, pathogenic and salutogenic forces must be in continually reciprocal relationship. In this region, in fact, our normal state can only arise by virtue of the fact that we swing back and forth, as it were, so as to paralyse, through stronger, health-giving forces, the pathogenic forces that are continually present; and, vice versa, oppose overburgeoning and potentially proliferative growth from the etheric realm with the limiting nature of the astral—which in turn leads to pathology if it exceeds its proper bounds and takes too strong a hold of the body. These facts relating to the thoracic organs are particularly important because they result, in fact, from a rhythm. This rhythm that arises is influenced, on the one hand, by everything occurring in the head, and on the other by all that occurs in metabolism. Therefore the cause of equilibrium in this essential rhythm really lies outside the chest itself, and we can say, in fact, that the human chest organs only, or chiefly, manifest effects. Causes of disorders there, for which we seek a cure, are not actually contained in the chest organs themselves. In a period, then, when human capacities of enquiry have become far removed from a more intuitive and direct grasp of things— as exemplified most brilliantly in the Viennese school of medicine, called 'nihilistic' because of its beliefs that one cannot go beyond pathology to arrive at therapy—such modern medical approaches have led, especially, to a gradual eradication of therapy and a sense that one can't get anywhere with it. The brilliance of this school is apparent, nevertheless, in the way it has promoted diagnosis of chest conditions and complaints.

Significant advances in the field of diagnosis of chest disorders arose here, with a prime emphasis on the advancement of knowledge yet with the least possible outcome of such knowledge—since this approach does not, at the same time, take other aspects of the human being into account. This is why so little is achieved, really—unless supplemented by other findings—by insight into what occurs in the human respiratory and circulatory organism alone. Naturally I would not suggest that such research is of little intrinsic value, but findings arising from, say, the stethoscope and suchlike, are only of major importance if complemented by understanding of the whole human being, so that one can then tackle things from a quite different perspective, making full use of what such a diagnosis can provide. Otherwise the findings of such a diagnosis are really only of academic interest. Of course one has to speak somewhat radically when addressing these issues in a contemporary way, but the truth of the matter underlies such radical formulations.

In recent times, disorders that specifically affect the chest have been distinguished by attempts to divert attention from the real issues, and resort instead to a somewhat mystical concept. While this concept does not have to remain mystical, it has certainly become so in the materialism of more recent times. Much has been made of 'endemic diseases' in relation to such disorders. Indeed, the idea of such 'endemic diseases' is clearly a large hold-all for everything that one does not wish to understand, and which in certain respects remains inaccessible to modern medical practice. Here I'll just highlight the rather interesting fact that the Viennese physician and professor Moritz Benedikt[9] conceived the—for him—somewhat strange idea of standing for election to the Austrian Parliament, backing up his candidacy by stating that his medical views compelled him to this step. This was, he said, because so many patients consulted him for whom he was unable to prescribe what he ought—that is, better clothing, habitation, better air and so forth. Such improvements, he went on, could only come about through social advances, and therefore, as a physician, he felt called upon to get involved in improving society. Here, in fact, one sees how the real problem is shifted elsewhere. Underlying all such things we find something that is of special importance for this aspect of the human being. You see, the pathological process developing in the human chest organism, and ultimately deriving from an irregularity in the interplay between astral and etheric, also has to be seen in such a context. Here we will make no further headway without insights gained by penetrating a little into the supersensible realm. And in relation to this the following has to be said.

The process of breathing unfolding between our outer surroundings and our inner organism is really one that cannot be understood at all if we do not grasp the nature of the astral realm. The distinctive reciprocal action there between oxygen and carbon is actually a continual interplay between the astral and the etheric. Now I beg you to consider that we normally spend a third of our life in a condition—that of sleep—where a large portion of our astral body exists outside the etheric body. And here you can see the important way in which the astral plays into human health. It is in fact self-evident that the astral is still active within us in sleep. Yet in this condition it no longer acts from the head but plays into us from the rest of the organism. During sleep the astral develops an activity which must remain behind in us in the right way even when the astral that has emerged through the head is outside us while we sleep.

Thus you see that simply by understanding the interplay between etheric and astral in conditions of health and disease in the human chest we can discover another rhythm unfolding in us—the rhythm of sleeping and waking. Actually, sleep itself, which as we will see is closely related to the process of metabolism, has less importance for the chest organs than it does for something else. And this other thing is, in turn, extraordinarily hard to detect. You may remember, if you were present at the time, the interesting range of symptoms we ascertained from use of substances with which we experimented here last time.[10] Dr Scheidegger demonstrated this on the board. But you will also recall that this array of symptoms consists of a great many isolated details, and that some skill is needed to compile and interrelate all these different symptoms. A difficulty may arise immediately when trying to form the right opinion about a condition in which, for example, you need to keep together the symptoms in the upper human being. If you then bring in a symptom which may be located in the upper human being but essentially is merely a symptom pushed up from metabolism you will be mistaken and this will give you the wrong idea about the whole situation. So we ought not to overlook how difficult it is, really, to ring-fence the details of a particular syndrome in the right way.

On the one hand it is certainly quite true to say that we can gradually acquire a correct, intuitive grasp of the relatedness of different symptoms within a syndrome. But on the other, while nature does help us, at the same time she makes it extremely hard for us to use the help she provides. In fact, nature unites and encompasses all the syndromes and does what we ourselves do when we formulate a comprehensive syndrome with all its divergent aspects. She does the same, but she makes it extraordinarily difficult for us to observe what she does. This is because she draws together the separate aspects of a syndrome in processes involved in falling asleep and waking—in the way we fall asleep and wake up again. What happens when someone falls asleep and wakes up again embodies nature's genius in drawing together aspects that come from different directions. However, physicians are of course very rarely in a position to base their understanding of this on anything other than what the patient tells them, which in most cases, and especially in the severest cases, will be imprecise. Of course we can carefully observe a patient as he falls asleep and wakes up, so that what the patient tells us—even if it seems to him to be the case—may then be of very little significance. If falling asleep and waking up are disturbed, the patient will of course tell us things about this process which, though living in his awareness, are unenlightening as far as a sound assessment is concerned. Here we have to look through and beyond what the patient relates. You can best recognize the truth of this if you try gradually to approach these facts and weigh them up carefully. Above all, you can experience the remarkable connection between the etheric and astral body if you observe how cares, worries and suchlike work on in people. Here it is not enough to observe the cares and anxieties that have occurred yesterday or in the past week, which are ultimately of least significance, but those which arose longer ago. A certain period must always elapse between the time when worries or griefs first affected someone, and the time when they have, in a sense, become organic, passing into the organism's activity. Cares and sorrows that reach a certain level of intensity always surface later on as anomalies in organic activity—and specifically in rhythmic organic activity. These may go as far as irregularities in the rhythmic organism; and only then can they work further to affect the metabolic organism and so forth. This is a primary fact that we have to consider. Above all, however improbable this appears to a materialistic view, we can also observe that hasty thinking, without awareness of why a person is thinking the thoughts he does, a kind of thinking in which one thought keeps elbowing another out of the way or follows immediately and compulsively on another's heels—a common and harmful trait of modern thinking—works on in the human organism after a certain period has elapsed, and does so in the rhythmic organism. This is an aspect of very great importance. Psychological processes should not be overlooked if we wish to understand abnormalities in the human rhythmic organism, notably what occurs in our chest organs. At the same time we can also include in this picture what we may call the periphery of the rhythmic organism: the rhythm of nutrition and of evacuation. By including the rhythm of nutrition and that of evacuation, we get a full picture of the overall rhythmic system.

On the other hand, something else is of very particular importance. The other pole of the human being, that of metabolism, works back on the rhythmic system, and we can perhaps best understand the way in which this occurs if we know the following: hunger and thirst manifest initially with great clarity in the human astral body. The way in which we ordinarily experience hunger and thirst is naturally as an astral phenomenon, astrally experienced awareness. We need to be quite clear about this. We ordinarily know nothing of whatever is not experienced astrally. What we experience etherically lies so far below in our subconscious that we are unaware of it. In daily life, therefore, hunger and thirst manifest in astral experience, but they cease to be astral in nature when they remain behind to be experienced under conditions of sleep. This does not mean, though, that they are then any less connected with the astral body that also works on in sleep, from below upwards. And what proceeds from this direction—hunger and thirst that work back on the rhythmic system when they remain in this way and work on within us—renders this system irregular by making it ill. This does not of course relate to the hunger and thirst we have felt the day before, which we take with us into sleep. It would be wrong to think that the problem arises when we go to sleep hungry now and then, or, if you like, when we go to sleep hungry over a longer period. That is not the harmful thing. What is harmful is for the state of hunger and thirst to become habitual, notably when this state is stimulated by a disorder of the metabolism so that the rest of the organism is not appropriately nourished in consequence. Thus the after-effects of hunger and thirst are, in this regard, certainly a cause underlying disorders of the respiratory and circulatory organism.

But if we now leave aside these effects on the human chest organs, the only other thing, a third factor, is the outer world's effect on us, for through breathing we are of course connected with the external world, and its effects unfold within us. Here, remarkably and importantly, a whole range of effects unfold in what is enclosed in the human ribcage, and partly also in the abdominal cavity, through the fact that rhythm reverberates there: effects from both our upper and lower organism along with effects from the outer world. A closer understanding of this rhythmic apparatus in us allows us to see that these effects unfold there; and we ourselves cannot remedy the causes that take effect there but must seek these causes elsewhere if we are to properly alleviate them. This is also why this region of the human being is so clearly the proper domain for the study of disease in general, and why, by starting here, our investigations must then trace their way further, work their way through to other areas.

The most striking and important realm of causes is really the one that lies outside us. For this rhythmic apparatus, engaged in the reciprocal action between oxygen and carbon, the chief astral influence basically lies in the external world. And here we need to discover how this apparatus connects and relates to the outer world. Spiritual-scientific enquiry shows the following: the earth *also* has a reciprocal relationship between what occurs below its surface—and here the term 'earth' certainly includes the actions of water—and what occurs above its surface. Basically a process so far inaccessible to mainstream scientists arises between the earth and its surroundings. And this process has aspects of extraordinary interest. An excellent way of studying it is by observing areas of the earth where this process of interplay between the earth and its surroundings is a very intimate one, and where much enters the earth's interior from outside it.

This is the case in the tropics. The distinctive nature of the tropical zone arises really from an intimate interplay between the external atmosphere—air, light and atmospheric heat—and what is contained within the earth itself. And it is also no accident that we must look there, in the tropics, for what I would call a certain pole of magnetic and electrical effects.

To speak metaphorically, of all areas of the earth the tropical zone is the one where most atmospheric effects are sucked up; and this imbibing of what exists outside the earth gives rise to burgeoning vegetation. Towards the poles, the earth sucks up little of these atmospheric effects, resisting them and as it were largely repulsing them. But in the tropics, if I can put it like this, the earth, seen from without, shines with least radiance because it reflects least back, being most absorbent there. At the poles, by contrast, the earth shines most, repulsing most of the external atmosphere and thus shining and gleaming with greatest radiance there.

This is extraordinarily important. By keeping this in mind we can gain insight into the fact, firstly, that at the tropics a great intimacy exists between etheric earth forces and atmospheric astral forces, whereas at the poles the astral is in a certain sense repulsed. By examining these circumstances further, however, such an insight can become very useful indeed. Let's assume we take a patient to a climate where the actions of light are very predominant, where the air is strongly illumined by light, suffused with it. If we do so we can discover that we have brought someone to a region where we can, basically, divert the earthly influences acting on him away from him, and expose him to influences coming from outside the earth. In strong sun effects, you see, there lies what the earth no longer uses or absorbs but is reflected back by it. So we take a patient to a region where he is exposed to these effects from outside the earth, and by doing so—by simply placing a patient in sun-illumined air—we work upon his rhythmic organism. And in fact we work in such a way that an irregular meta-bolism is directly combated by rhythm due to the latter itself being naturally regulated by such exposure to light.

These are circumstances that lead us to understand the real basis of sun and light cures. And if someone has greatly lowered resistance to parasitic infections, a cure of this kind would be highly recommended. We don't have to subscribe to the bacillus theory but just have to realize that the presence of parasites has deeper causes, which allow the bacilli to accumulate and persist. The bacilli themselves are never the real pathogens, but merely show us that a patient contains these 'pathogens' within him. Bacillus research is important, certainly, but only as the basis of further enquiry, for the real organic causes of an illness lie in the human being himself. These organic causes within us are counteracted by what rays towards the earth from the surrounding cosmos, and what surrounds but is not wholly absorbed by the earth. Thus it is an excess energy, a superfluity of sun, light and so forth. In other words, where the earth no longer only sprouts and burgeons with vegetation but where it begins to shine and gleam; where, therefore, it contains light in excess of what it needs to sprout and burgeon, we have something of very beneficial effect in this regard.

The following is also particularly beneficial here. If we find that a patient is particularly susceptible to parasitic infections due to an irregular circulatory organism, it is a very good idea—of course first considering all other circumstances, a wide range of which we will meet in subsequent lectures—to take him to a higher altitude than the one he is used to, a greater altitude above sea level, and thus give him an 'altitude cure'. And such altitude cures—which of course can be harmful in other circumstances for, as we saw yesterday, everything beneficial in one instance can be harmful in another—will have a beneficial effect on conditions of this type. Now, though, we need to consider something else. We must not forget what is present in certain artificially synthesized substances I referred to previously, or the effects of these on people exposed to them, which we first need to evaluate. By 'artificially synthesized substances' I mean here substances and foods we do not merely consume as the given fruits of nature but which we cook or in some other way prepare for introduction into our organism, for instance through combustion and then intake of the ash residue or suchlike. Here we ourselves subject an earthly substance to a process which really incorporates effects external to the earth. Cooking and combustion do indeed raise out of the earthly domain whatever is cooked or combusted. So by giving cooked or combusted substances to a person, we give rise in him to an inner effect that is similar to allowing increased sunlight or the climate of a higher altitude to work upon him. We will also need to consider how we might now be in a position to encourage someone, on the one hand, to change his diet in a certain way, and on the other also administer a particular medicine to him. This is in cases where an irregular rhythmic system becomes apparent. At all events we must certainly consider whether we need to give him a substance that has arisen through combusting something of vegetable origin, for by combusting vegetable substance we surpass and outdo the normal vegetable process. Through combustion we extend the process with something that comes from outside the earth.

Then the following is also especially important: phenomena involving electricity and magnetism encompass a process on earth or a sum of processes on earth which are inwardly connected with what we must call both earthly and non-earthly. The field of electricity and magnetism is one which really ought to be studied more deeply in relation to human health and illness. Here, though, we should feel our way very carefully due to the following: if you picture the surface of the earth to yourself schematically (see Fig. 9)—here the interior of the earth, and here what is above it—then phenomena of electricity and magnetism have a close connection to what is intrinsically earthly in nature. [See also Plate 3]

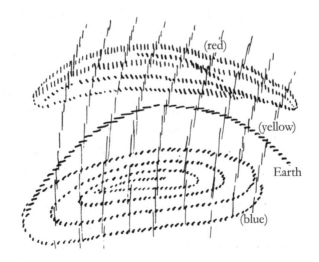

(red)

(yellow)

Earth

(blue)

Fig. 9

You know of course that electricity conducts itself from one earth conductor to another, say from one morse telegraph station to the next: there is only ever one wire connection and the circuit is completed underground. Here we see the electrical field which the earth has already appropriated. We can say that electricity and magnetism are basically constituted by something that is both outside the earth and within it (yellow). But the earth appropriates electricity and contains electrical effects that really originate outside of the earth (blue). In fact the electrical and also magnetic effects can be held back in the earth's atmospheric periphery (red) without being appropriated by the earth. These are all the electrical and magnetic effects which we find in our electrical and magnetic fields.

If we magnetize iron, in relation to the earth this means we turn the magnet into a little thief. We endow it with the capacity to rob the earth and retain what the latter wishes to absorb from the cosmos, before it can do so. Thus we make the magnet into a little robber. It appropriates what the earth wants and has the inward strength to retain it for itself. All electrical and magnetic fields we have created on the earth are really stolen from the earth for our own use; and thus we inveigle nature into stealing, teach it to keep beyond the earth's reach what comes from outside the earth. And here we have something eminently extraterrestrial, which we cunningly retain above the earth although the earth seeks with all its strength to draw it inside itself, in order to let it stream out from itself again. But we do not allow it to do so, holding it back instead from this activity. And this is why we must regard electrical and magnetic fields as excellent opponents of arrhythmic processes in us. Thus really a form of therapy should be developed which specifically addresses severe arrhythmia or any other severe or mild disorders of the rhythmic system—in mild cases it works even better—by holding a strong magnet close to the human organism, not actually touching the body, at a distance that would need to be determined experimentally. You would have to try this out to get the right distance.

Further to this, I'd like to suggest how one might best use our scientific findings not so much in order to communicate an interesting fact—one not yet far enough developed to pass on to mainstream science—but to draw your attention to something which can guide and govern a quite different train of thought.

The same Professor Benedikt whom I spoke of earlier has undertaken very interesting experiments in a darkroom on the radiance of human auras.[11] These experiments have nothing directly to do with what I described for instance in the book *Theosophy,* although there is an indirect connection. The emanations I described can only be perceived supersensibly. But between these higher emanations and the coarser ones which the ordinary eye can detect lies a field that can be perceived in the darkroom; and Professor Benedikt has provided an interesting account of what he found under darkroom conditions. For his experimental subjects he chose, in particular, people who were sensitive to dowsing rod phenomena—in whose hands, in other words, the dowsing rod responded most actively. Moriz Benedikt tested the auras of such people in the darkroom, and found the following very interesting results: that the auras of people with a skill in dowsing are quite different from those of others. To be precise, the asymmetry of the former is very pronounced so that the aura of their left side behaves in quite a different way from their right. The aura emanating from their head is also quite different. Though these results were greeted sceptically, they represent the beginning of recording the human aura through physical demonstrations. We must be clear however that such phenomena are only of the lowest kind, and connected with our physical organization. The sphere of supersensible perception is not yet involved here, as some, who wish easy access to it, would like to claim. But it is nevertheless a beginning that could lead to a therapeutic outcome. One might investigate what happens by applying a strong magnet to the back of someone, say, with incipient tuberculosis—thus allowing such a person to be irradiated by a magnetic field, and enhancing this action by moving the magnet, held crosswise, from above downwards and from below upwards. In this way the whole chest organism would gradually be suffused by the magnetic field. In applying this magnetic field one does not need a light field too, at the same time, for this would only disrupt the effect. So you see one could perfectly well place a patient in a darkroom and could soon perceive distinct emanations proceeding from his fingers. Having done this, placing the patient in the darkroom and

applying a strong magnet to his back and perceiving the subtle emanations from his fingertips—whose form will be that of a cone with
outward-pointing tip—we can be sure that the patient has really been
suffused or irradiated with a magnetic field. You will find that this has a
range of extremely beneficial effects for combating disorders such as
those implicated in tuberculosis of the lungs.

At the same time, such things demonstrate the great importance of
remembering the principle that we really only have effects in the human
chest; and that therefore, when we wish to bring about a cure, we must
turn to our surroundings and use something that belongs to the world
external to us: light, climatic influences, taking a patient to a higher
altitude and every aspect of the magnetic field. This is true too of the
electrical field, but here we must give special consideration to the mode
of treatment involved. Placing an electrical pole directly on the human
organism and allowing electricity to pass through it is quite a different
matter from first creating an electrical field and placing a person into
this field without a circuit passing directly through him from one pole to
the other. It will be necessary to experiment with such things, which are
extraordinarily important. Under certain circumstances one can also
obtain beneficial effects by allowing the circuit to pass between two
poles through a person. But the action in this case will only be one that
works over from the metabolic into the rhythmic system. When I
conduct electricity through a person, passing it from one pole to the
other and as it were including the person in the electrical circuit, only
the metabolic system is affected. If, on the other hand, I place him into
an electrical field, I will notice everywhere on him the same kinds of
emanation as were found in the darkroom experiments—pointed rays
on toes and fingers and so forth—and I will find that I can treat patients
by this means, even those whose digestion and so forth is well regulated
but who show tuberculosis-related disorders. This is particularly relevant for disorders that arise in this area.

Today, therefore, we were concerned initially with our external surroundings. I have drawn your attention to how, in sleeping and waking,
nature brings together what is otherwise distributed separately across a
range of symptoms. Tomorrow I will come back to this, first showing
the diagnostic importance of the moment of falling asleep, and of

awakening, but at the same time also examining how we can observe what nature tries to intimate to us in our waking up and falling asleep. Then however, as long as we are aware of this principle, we can use it to regulate observation of our syndromes, and will find in particular that this can also give us an important pointer to the different forms of treatment required in addressing chronic and acute illnesses.

LECTURE 4

DORNACH, 14 APRIL 1921

YESTERDAY I said that certain syndromes are encompassed in the phenomena of falling asleep and waking up. Initially it is of primary importance to consider the symptoms comprised in the process of falling asleep, and here the following must be stated: difficulties in falling asleep always indicate that the astral body—I will use this term here since you are now all very familiar with it—clings to the physical and etheric organs, especially the latter, and is too strongly connected to them. A spiritual investigator can easily detect how the astral body clings on in this way by the fact that the organs, both physical and others, continue to function as they do during waking life, whereas in normal conditions of falling asleep they undergo a marked decline in activity.

I said yesterday that it is very difficult, of course, to properly assess the full scope and significance of such sleep-related phenomena. We therefore need to acquire a comprehensive view, as it were, of the phenomena which in a waking state are concomitant with difficulties in falling asleep. We find such concomitant phenomena in all that, in a certain way, points to involuntary function of the organism. In other words, any involuntary twitching of the lips or blinking of the eyelids, any excessive movement of the fingers and suchlike, anything in fact that does not give expression to an inner process, and thus all sorts of fidgeting, is indicative in waking life of a reduced capacity to fall asleep. Naturally we can mostly only detect this process when it is clearly apparent externally. When such twitching occurs in relation to our internal organs, we will need to acquire a certain skill in detecting it, and learn how to properly connect certain symptoms. For instance, one can detect certain noises in patients suffering from chlorosis, in the blood vessels descending on the left and right side of the neck and further down. Such noises, formerly called 'venous hum' (I am not sure if this is still the term used for them) can be detected in all of us if we turn the head abruptly to the left or right—when, in other words, we initiate a strong development of astrality, which always occurs if we carry out involuntarily a movement usually otherwise voluntary. Astrality is exerted too strongly, used too strongly, pushed too strongly towards an organ every time that a movement usually carried out voluntarily—thus a movement dependent on the I—becomes involuntary, and thereby acquires a twitchy quality. By indirect observations of this kind we can learn to detect twitching in the inner organs.

Problems falling asleep always indicate an irregularity somewhat inaccessible to direct external medical interventions. This irregularity is far removed from phenomena I described yesterday in relation to such things as light, and magnetic and electrical fields. All that is concomitant with difficulty in falling asleep is somewhat removed from such phenomena, and here, therefore, we must resort to medicines. Thus if we find a syndrome that can be summarized as 'problems in falling asleep', medicines will be needed, specifically ones involving processes induced by cooking or combusting vegetable substances. Where we find problems in falling asleep and disorders of the human thorax—and thus a condition involving the astral body's over-adherence to physical and etheric organs—all medicines obtained by decocting roots and by ashing or combustion will be of great importance. All the strength concentrated in a root decoction and plant ash will play an especially important role here. On the other hand, everything I described yesterday will be of most significance where there is a difficulty in waking up.

Poor capacity to wake from sleep always indicates that the astral body is engaging too little with the organs. In chest disorders, this reduced engagement of the astral body has a somewhat different significance compared with general illnesses of the human organism. In the latter case one has to try to induce the whole astral body to enter more strongly. Then what I said a few days ago about the effects of arsenic comes into its own. This is only effective, though, when it is a matter of treating an astral body already permeated by the I. If one needs to treat the astral body alone, in contrast, it will be of particular importance to resort to the kinds of measure I described yesterday. Difficulty in waking up is always accompanied by symptoms one can describe as a dazed state or a tendency for consciousness to remain dulled. In other words, the symptoms accompanying difficulties in waking up after sleep are largely mental or psychological ones. For those patients, therefore, who show any impairment of their chest organism and who, at the same time, manifest accompanying psychological symptoms of this kind, it will be very important to use cures involving magnetic or electrical fields as I described. Here, though, I would like to note the following in response to a question I was asked yesterday. (As far as time allows I will try to respond to all questions put to me during these lectures.) The question related to the difference between treatment with direct current and alternating current. If a patient is clearly in a frail condition, suffering for example from malnutrition and so forth—so that the disorder proceeds more from what I will call the lower part of the middle organism—it is better to use alternating current. If, on the other hand, it is clear that a disorder proceeds from the upper organism, it will be better to use direct current. However, the difference is not very great, and you will not go far wrong by using either.

You will have gathered that precisely in this area of human health and illness one also finds important points of reference for general dietary measures. A subtle transition exists here between effects of a more dynamic nature, externally applied, and those arising from plant substances we first process and transform ourselves. But you will understand that because we are considering the region in us where everything relies on rhythm, on rhythmic functioning in the human organism, something else also arises here which is essential to consider when assessing health and sickness: that our approach must avoid fanaticism of all kinds. The kind of fanaticism which can come to expression, say, in extreme forms of raw food diets, applied fanatically as dietary prescription, will have a very specific consequence for the whole human organism. Raw food—in other words never eating in cooked form the parts of a plant that are lower down, towards the root—means that the health of the respiratory system is gradually undermined. The human organism isn't easily wrecked and so the ruinous effects of a fanaticism of this kind will not become apparent for a long time. Gradually, though, an extreme raw food diet will express itself in marked shortness of breath or similar conditions.

Yet someone might come along and object that they had excellent results with a fruit diet. Then the following must be said. Fruits are not roots, but are strongly exposed to external sun. Here a pronounced extraterrestrial process is accomplished that comes very close to cooking and draws on the dynamic potential in fruit. Thus if certain patients are given fresh fruit, specifically not roots, this will do a great deal less harm than letting them eat uncooked roots. We must not be fanatical in either direction but instead find an individualized approach that can go both ways. There may very well be cases where it becomes clearly apparent that the irregularity in a person's chest system originates in his circulation and not in the respiratory rhythm. If I can be sure that the disorder originates in the circulation and not the respiratory rhythm I will need to turn to something that plays over from the digestive functions into the circulatory functions; and here I will make up for what is lacking by giving a diet of raw fruit. That will be absolutely right—in such a case one can certainly resort to a raw fruit diet. But if impairment of chest function tends to originate in a patient's breathing, such treatment will achieve nothing and may even be harmful. Here, instead, I will need to provide a diet of cooked roots. The instability of fluctuating dynamics in this system shows clearly how misplaced any particular form of fanaticism is.

Now we will not gain a full understanding of this system, and will therefore have to cover the same ground again, if we do not take account in this first part of our course—which focuses more on pathology, whereas the second part will focus more on therapy—of a process in the human organism that is very often entirely inaccessible to external observation, and whose deleterious effect on human health therefore remains unobserved. In my general lectures, in speaking of philology[12] (though this theme could equally well have figured in the section on science) I spoke of remarkable processes that discharge outwards from the organism at puberty, whereas they discharge inwards in the period between birth and the change of teeth—when a child is learning to talk therefore. The processes that occur here between the human astral body and etheric body, and also the physical body, underlie the acquisition of speech in a child and all the changes in the human organism connected with this. We should therefore observe these processes very carefully in a child. As he learns to talk this always goes hand in hand with changes in the rest of the organism. And as I said, we ought also to trace back these changes in reverse, towards birth, in other words looking back from the radical reconfiguration at second dentition to the time when the child was learning to talk. But now we find an equally important change that is more inward-directed and is not so outwardly apparent as, for instance, second dentition—which anyone will notice—or learning to speak. We will likewise all be aware of the child's developing speech, which manifests outwardly. This other change is almost more important for health and illness than the others—which, as I said, are palpable and apparent and therefore engage what I will call our instinctive educational actions. A much greater significance underlies this other, more hidden process, which occurs in the period between the change of teeth and puberty, right in the middle of this period. Here the true I—which is really only exoterically born, as I have said elsewhere, born in a fully exoteric way, around the age of 20—is born into the child, just as the astral body is born in the acquisition of speech. This process culminates between the age of eight and nine.

And now please consider the following. Our I-related predisposition, the I-capacity in us, is scarcely ever taken into account. Indwelling the human organism, the I does something very particular. Everything else in us, our physical attributes—which we will certainly return to in detail—our etheric, and also astral level of existence, which really only enters into connection with the outside world through oxygen, are aspects of our being that are very strongly connected to our interior. Almost alone amongst the aspects of the human organism, the astral body is withdrawn from us in sleep by the I. The astral body has a very strong affinity with the physical body and even more so with the etheric body. But this is not true of the I. And here, notably in the relationship and connection of the I with the outer world, we see the profound difference between the human being and the animal. When we ingest food we absorb substances that are also external substances, and must be transformed within us. Who causes this transformation, this thorough transformation of outer substances within us? Who does this? In truth, it is the I. The I alone has the power of, as it were, extending its feelers down into the forces of external substances. [See Plate 4, top] If you have an external substance—I'll draw it schematically like this—it has certain forces that have to be separated out if they are to be recombined in the human organism. Etheric body and astral body in a certain sense tiptoe round the substances, and do not have the strength to penetrate their inner nature: they just circle round them. Only the I really engages in penetrating the substances themselves and delving into them. So when you offer a food substance to the human organism, this food is first inside us. The I however reaches beyond the whole human organism and directly enters the food substance. Thus a reciprocal action arises between the inner forces of the food substance and the human I. Here the outer world, in respect of chemistry and physics, and the internal world of the human being, in respect of anti-chemistry and anti-physics, extend into each other. That is the important thing.

Up to the time when the second teeth begin to develop, thus the beginning of second dentition, this engagement with food substances is governed from the head. The child has been constituted during foetal development so that at birth he has received forces via his head that are active in assimilating substances from within. But after second dentition, in the time leading up to puberty, and culminating between the ninth and tenth year, the I that works from our lower organism, the lower I, has to meet and engage with the upper I. In children the I always acts from the upper organism to assimilate substances, until the age referred to. I mean of course the instruments of the I. The I itself is ultimately a unified entity. But the I's instruments—the polarity of I activity expressed in the lower I which meets the upper I—only establish a proper mutual relationship at this age between the ninth and tenth year. The I has to enter the human organization in the same way as the astral body must engage with the human organization when a child learns to speak.

With these considerations in mind, let us now observe everything that becomes apparent in children from the eighth or ninth year onwards through to the age of eleven or twelve—aspects that are so important to take account of in children's schooling at this age. Starting from the perspective I have outlined, we will find the outer expression of these phenomena in a search in which the human organism is engaged—which involves searching for a harmony established only during the course of life between assimilated substances and our inner organization. Try to observe carefully how the head at this age does not much want to assimilate substances' inner forces, how it objects to this, and how this comes to expression in headaches around the ninth, tenth or eleventh year. Then observe how concomitant conditions arise in metabolic disorders, ones that manifest relatively close to the exterior, in the secretion of gastric acid and so forth. If you observe all these things you can see how some children are continually ailing, in a sense, due to this lack of adjustment between the I acting from below and from above. If we pay careful attention to such things we can remedy them, and after puberty they will normally fade and vanish; for at this age the astral body catches up and can compensate for what the I is not able to accomplish. These things gradually diminish from the fourteenth or fifteenth year through to the twentieth or twenty-first. Children ailing at this period between second dentition and puberty can later become extraordinarily healthy, and it is very instructive to observe this. You will often have seen how ailing children, especially those in whom this sickliness expresses itself in digestive disorders, in irregular digestion, later go on to flourish and be fully healthy when carefully treated. It is very important that such treatment should take great care in relation to dietary prescriptions. Wonderful things can be achieved as long as the parents or teachers of children with this kind of ailment refrain from continually offering large amounts of food which they try to persuade them to eat. This will continually exacerbate the condition. Instead we should try to discover what the child can easily digest, what he can assimilate especially well; and then we should serve this to him in smaller, more frequent portions, thus distributing food intake over a larger number of meals. This will do these children a great deal of good. It is quite mistaken to think we are achieving anything by over-feeding, persuasion and suchlike. If, in addition, we ensure that such children are not too overburdened by schoolwork—which will increasingly exacerbate their condition—but instead give them enough rest and leisure, we will also be enhancing the inwardly necessary digestive activity achieved by offering smaller portions of food. The very opposite of this is done on a large scale, and by overlooking or transgressing this law we do not nurture healthy human development. Instead, all sorts of predispositions for illness potentially result from these digestive ailments, and can continue to affect a person for the rest of his life.

In the Waldorf School[13] people are quick to complain that we give children so little homework. There are good reasons for this. An educational approach in tune with reality does not just uphold abstract principles, or the general abstractions often proposed today, but instead takes account of everything that needs to inform a person's actual development. Above all this includes not overburdening children with homework, which can sometimes, certainly, be the deeply concealed cause of poor digestion. Such things always only manifest later in life, but they are real factors. Remarkably, supersensible insight into human development can show us how conditions that only come to the fore later in life are already apparent in hints and signs at an earlier age.

A danger lies in what I will call the engagement or coupling of the lower I with the human organism. It exists really for all people, and poses a particular risk for children in modern civilization. Anyone not of sturdy peasant stock should be aware of this risk. A strong distinction still exists in relation to such things, and must be made here, between people of peasant or farming stock and the rest of us. All the rest of the world's population has a very marked predisposition to risks arising from this insufficient engagement of the I with the organism, which is thoroughly ruined before this I is due to engage it. Such risks appear as the I engages from below. In the respiratory system and also the head system, the female constitution is more susceptible to this remarkably unstable balance. Men are more robust—though not more stable—in relation to their chest organization, and therefore less sensitive or susceptible. While the same problems can affect them, these are likely to be less apparent. The female sex is more sensitive to everything that occurs here; and what I have described as the search for the right kind of engagement or coupling of the I either culminates in a healthy condition or in anaemia. Anaemia is the direct continuation of all abnormal occurrences of this kind after the age of seven. It only surfaces later as a disorder, but represents an intensification of factors that are present but unnoticeable at an earlier stage of life.

Here we must make an extremely important distinction. In considering the circulatory system we must distinguish circulation itself, as a sum of motions, from what in turn intimately informs this circulation and as it were penetrates it, which is metabolism. The circulatory system is informed by an equilibrium between the metabolic system and the rhythmic system, whereas the respiratory system reveals an equilibrium between the rhythmic organism and the organism of nerves and senses. Observing this middle realm of the human organism, the chest system, we have to remember that it is organized between two polarities. Through breathing it is organizationally related to the head, and through circulation to the system of metabolism and limbs. Everything in the metabolism itself or in what intimately accompanies the metabolism as our capacity for movement—which is of great importance especially in the first or 'rising' half of life—pushes its way into the circulatory forces as forces of metabolism. And this upward-pushing dynamic must in turn advance so that, in the process I described, we find that what the I brings about in metabolism and also in the assimilation of substances advances into strong engagement with the substances' inner forces. We find here an upward migration through circulation and breathing that extends as far as the head system, and this has to organize itself properly in the period I spoke of between second dentition and sexual maturity. The I's capacity to grasp hold of, to engage with, the forces of external substances, must migrate upwards through circulation and breathing until it acts properly upon the head system. This is the very complex process we have to study; and we can really only do so by trying to understand its effect in what I would call the outer digestive tract—where substances still strongly resemble the form they have in the outer world and where our inner processes have as yet taken only a weak hold of them. What is this first engagement with external substances, in fact? What is the I doing when it first grasps hold of external substance?

When the I first grasps the forces of external substances this is accompanied by taste sensations, taste, the assimilation of outer substances in the subjective experience of tasting. This is the first engagement of our inner forces. Then the process works its way inward. But tasting also extends inwards. The inner digestive organism—in other words on the other side of the intestine, leading over into the blood—is still an attenuated tasting. And really this continues upwards, until tasting is countered in the head. Here tasting is deadened. The head opposes and deadens the process of tasting, which must, though, first fully unfold. The I naturally takes stronger hold of substances, penetrates them more deeply than is the case in mere outward, subjective tasting.

What occurs, in a sense, in the external digestive tract is strongly influenced by the mineral or salt element. Every aspect of what I am saying now accords with my expositions in the previous course, and, as you will see, mostly extends and enlarges on it. The fact of the matter is as follows. A basic and essential question in medicine is to ask what a medicament actually is. What is a medicine, derived as it is from the outer realm of nature?

Whatever the organism can digest when healthy is not a medicine. This cannot be a medicine. We can only start to speak of a medicine when we administer something to the organism which it cannot digest when healthy, which must therefore only be assimilated in an abnormal human organism. We challenge the abnormal human organism to assimilate something that is not assimilated in a healthy human organism. Healing is therefore a continuation of digestion—but digestion, in fact, which is gradually transposed into the interior of the human organism.

The most palpable and fully developed forms of, say, anaemia are accompanied by the following concomitant symptoms: tiredness, lethargy, difficulty in falling asleep or in waking up. Given all these symptoms, which can affect most children between second dentition and puberty, we first have to try to remedy the condition in the external digestive tract. Here we have to use mineral substance, still entirely mineral in character.[14] And we will find this to be beneficial. Initially these things may be observed as symptoms, strong symptoms, which all indicate how the I is seeking to grasp hold outwardly of the forces of external substances, and how it can be supported in this endeavour by, say, carbonated iron. Iron carbonate is something that supports the organism in combating lethargy whenever the I needs to get an outward grip.

If we take this a stage further, we find the I intervening too weakly in the circulatory organism. Then we will see how the I's lack of engagement in the circulatory organism can, for example, be supported by Ferrum muriaticum,[15] thus by a medicine enhanced and intensified in the purely mineral realm.

If we continue to the respiratory organism, thus advancing another stage higher, we can give very particular support to the I by using vegetable acid. Rising further, to the head system, we can do this with the pure metals—not of course as pure metals in an external sense, for initially these have no proper relationship to the human organism, but instead in their subtlest powers. This is why I said last year that basically the human organism won't let you muck about with it by using metals allopathically, for it is itself a homoeopath. In the ascent from the digestive system to the head organism, it fragments the metals itself— and we can of course support the organism in this process by potentizing a substance.

But you will find—and we will return to this later and look at it from a different angle—that we can learn something here about potentiza- tion. We have to ascertain the actual locus of the deficiency. The lower and further away from the head the deficiency or lack of engagement is centred in the human organism, the lower should be the potencies we use. The nearer we find it to be to the head organization, the higher are the potencies required. It is of course the case that what comes too close to the head organization can express itself in all sorts of ways.

How the I grasps hold of the external world is a real point of departure which will enable us to fathom the symptomatic phenomena we encounter. If you reflect on the things we have been discussing over the past few days, you will recall my emphasis on a view of the human organism that cannot be encompassed in terms of shapes and outlines—

for these only represent solid tissue. The human organism is largely also organized fluid, organized air and organized temperature. And now, you see, the I has to engage and grasp hold of these different aspects of the organism. Especially important, and subtle in nature, is the engagement of the I in the body's different temperature conditions. The I has to engage in these temperature variations within the body in the following way.

At birth we have an image of the I. The image or imprint of the I is present in the head, as stated previously. The I is present there as image and works throughout childhood. And now, alongside this, the I must as it were give reality or existence from below, must engage in the organism. This is expressed in the fact that this image of the I we have in our head permeates our organism with warmth in childhood, is connected with the warming of the human organism. However, this permeation with warmth fades—it is strongest at birth in so far as the warming process issues from the head, and then falls away. [See Plate 4] And later on in life we need to maintain at a peak, from below, the warmth that develops in this way, and to do so through the engagement of the I in these temperature conditions. As we grow older we have to oppose this lapsing graph of warmth with the other, rising one, which largely depends on a capacity to grasp hold of rising forces made available from food substance, and to lead these into circulation, breathing and the head system.

Now let us assume that this does not happen in the proper way, that there is insufficient strength to assimilate the inner forces of external substances into the human organism. Let us assume this is too weak, and is not developed with adequate intensity. In that case you are not, as you should, introducing enough warmth into the organism via the I. The head, developing only the declining graph of warmth, allows the body to grow too cold. This becomes apparent firstly at the extremities. So please observe, now, how the state of flagging energy derived from all I described today is intensified in such people—in symptoms of chilled hands and toes. This is very tangible, for you can feel here how the process that was accomplished in childhood from above downwards through the image of the I is not adequately met or countered with what needs to arise from and be developed by the active I, which should carry warmth through into the furthest extremities of the limbs. This is something that will show you how, as soon as you see things in images, as soon as you take note of how the different powers above and below are subtly interacting so that images arise, developing into something as fine and subtle as pictorial quality, then, in what comes to expression there we really have what I would call images. In chilled hands and feet you find images of what is occurring in the whole human organism. And then we can learn to assess the symptoms in a way that allows knowledge of the whole human being to leap out at us from them. If a person has chilled hands and feet this is profoundly indicative of a failure of this I to engage properly in later life. If we take account of such things, or if in general we simply engage with what spiritual science has to say, based on its fundamental approach, we can forge a real connection with the human organism. A failure to do this, to take account of such things, will gradually lead to a loss of connection and capacity to really perceive and understand the human organism. If we engage with what spiritual science has to offer, on the other hand, we acquire a connection with and insight into the human organism. We grow into it.

Take the following example. This spiritual science continually stresses that there is something intrinsic in the power which enables us to stand upright, and that this power is in turn connected with the development of the I from below upwards. What first happens when we learn to raise ourselves upright expresses a power of uplift which is in a certain sense only external. It is supported by what streams down from above. Once the change of teeth has been completed, the power to raise ourselves has correspondingly used itself up: this primary power of uplift has come to a conclusion and then the self-raising energy passes into our interior, where a balance must be created between what rises from below upwards and what streams from above downwards. And then the forces coming from above and those coming from below enter into mutual opposition, encounter each other. In this one-dimensional encounter, as I will call it, of the forces from above and those from below, we can see particularly well what is happening at this age. And now observe how people with, say, chlorosis or anaemia grow very tired. They do not feel most tired when they walk on level ground but when they're climbing stairs. This points us directly to these phenomena.

People with a tendency to anaemia are especially taxed by climbing stairs; and so, in such symptoms, and in what comes to living expression as a child grows, we can grasp hold of spiritual realities underlying our existence. And then we can come to the point of simply 'reading off' what we need to do to remedy abnormal conditions from what diagnostic pathology can tell us in this way. We will speak further of this tomorrow.

LECTURE 5

THESE observations will culminate in a description of the nature of the medicines we have assembled and which should then be brought into wider circulation. However, we will not be able to speak properly about the knowledge and skill necessary for using these medicines without the full preparation that is still required. Today, therefore, we will consider several aspects that can lead us into the whole fabric of the human being, as this develops and emerges through the interplay of I, astral body, etheric body and physical body. I have mentioned already that, through a particular action of arsenic, it is possible to induce the astral body to enter further into the organs than is otherwise the case in a particular patient, and that this astral body of course draws the I into or with it.

Now, drawing the astral body more into the organs increases their mineralizing process; and therefore we can also say that where we notice the organs as such are too strongly vitalized, are developing excessive life forces, and in a sense proliferating etherically, then we can heal this condition by administering arsenic. If we wish to, we can also even describe what happens inwardly in such a condition in terms of an external process, which has what we might call an elective affinity with the process in the human being. To express this affinity of the astral body with the etheric body, and via the latter with the physical body, we could certainly coin the term 'arsenize'. A mild arsenizing process continually takes place in us, and is present in most pronounced form at the moment we wake up. We must be clear that the human organism certainly has the quality of the metal in it as a system of forces. This elective affinity certainly exists between the human being and the surrounding earth and cosmos: certain processes occur in us that occur outside us too, and, for example, come to conclusion and rest in the metals. When we speak of an arsenization process in us, therefore, we should not imagine that arsenic itself is directly active there but rather that our inner activity works in the same way as arsenic does in the external world. And thus we can gain insight into how we must aid and support such activity within us. If, therefore, you consider this arsenizing—which one might also call astralizing—of the human organism, you will be able to discover that when this activity is too strong it can manifest in a rise in temperature in the stomach region, and even in a certain ease of digestion and assimilation—but this can in fact be cause for concern if it becomes too easy, since all such easing within us is followed in turn by reactions and greater problems. All this is connected with a certain mineralization within us. It is possible to investigate and confirm this, though it must be done in the right way— that is, by taking all other factors into account as well. For instance, the corpses of people who strongly astralize, and in whose organic, physical processes arsenization is therefore at work, will decay less easily than those in whom the astral body is too weakly connected with the organs. This is certainly something we should take note of. In extreme form we can see it in the tendency to mummification of corpses poisoned by arsenic. They mummify and show strong resistance to the process of decay.

Now we must ask how we can counter an excessive arsenizing or astralizing process in a person when, if you like, he is becoming mummified while still alive. It is necessary to connect an observation, a way of looking, with such a condition. If someone is becoming too strongly mummified, what can we do to counter this? To put it radically, we temporarily turn him into a tooth. This will help us trace some of the mysterious workings of the human organism. We make the whole human being into a tooth: in other words, taking the whole organism into account we try in some way to administer to him the radiant power of magnesium, magnesium in some medicinal form. The radiant power of magnesium described by Professor Roemer[16] is then invoked through the whole organism; and this points us really very clearly towards a relationship which exists between the astral body—including and encompassing the I within it—on the one hand, and the etheric body and physical body on the other.

Now let us try to look at the opposite picture, a condition where the astral body with the I tends to penetrate the organs too little; and in which therefore the organs start to be left to their own devices in so far as they are provided for by physical and etheric activity. This is a condition that manifests when there is no proper reciprocity of nutrition, in the mutual interaction between our surroundings and our inner, organic processes. The inner, organic processes start energetically developing their own vital energy, and cease to be receptive to outside influence. The powers of the I no longer penetrate food substances so thoroughly, and in consequence the astral body is also engaged one-sidedly, and cannot gain proper access to the etheric body. What I would call a proliferation of physical and etheric activity occurs, initially manifesting as diarrhoea, and concomitant signs such as blood in the stool. Inner vital activity can become so strong that small pieces of organic tissue separate from the intestinal walls and are excreted in the stool. The stool itself may even become a serum-type fluid, a strong indication that vital energy within is proliferating without hindrance from the astralizing forces. Such things occur. Finally, even protein is carried along by this process and excreted without being properly assimilated. Conditions of this nature ultimately point to a failure of astral body and I to work into our physical and etheric levels as they must, to accomplish these semi-conscious motions necessary for the human organism. Picture this now: the astral body and I are not engaged here in the right way, and thus the etheric body and physical forces are left to their own devices, giving rise to tenesmus, which is characteristic of such conditions. The more this state of affairs pertains, the more that normal conditions of diarrhoea progress to dysentery and beyond; and thus the further you proceed in describing this pathology, the more you will see that it must be described in a way that invokes the picture opposite to that of arsenizing or astralizing processes. Everywhere you will find the counter-image of astralization or arsenization. And since the astral body is strongly involved here, you will be led more or less naturally to the conclusion that the medicine needed to combat this disorder derives from arsenic—that in other words arsenization is required to counteract such conditions.

I believe that it can enormously enrich and intensify our ideas here if we realize that, basically, everything that occurs within us finds its correspondence in processes outside us in the surrounding world. And even if such things evidently sound repugnant to someone who has undergone conventional training, I will not refrain from using certain expressions—as long as we understand them in the right way—that have real meaning for spiritual science and can thoroughly ground us in these realities.

What we can observe in the human being as the process of arsenizing, astralizing, or if you like the way the physical organism becomes brittle or mummified, is basically exactly the same process as occurs in rock formation. Wherever the earth forms rocks, it is in a sense poisoned or beginning to be poisoned by arsenic. By contrast imagine that the external astrality which surrounds the earth everywhere—as I pointed out in the last lecture course—in a sense bypasses the earth's surface, bypasses this external astrality's task of bringing forth blossoms and drawing plants from the soil to the sphere above ground, and succeeds in penetrating below the earth's surface. Imagine that it bypasses the earth and adheres to water—and then, in such regions, the earth gets dysentery. When the external, cosmic astrality works or is able to work on groundwater, the earth gets dysentery. This process I am describing is one based on reality, underpinned by many real factors, and we should attend to it carefully, for it can give us insight into the connection between what happens below the earth's surface and disorders such as dysentery. We can often discern in such things a kind of sub-earthly effect, from the watery realm, on the human being. The important thing here will be to take account of the astral body's strong involvement and to realize in consequence that we will need to use medium doses, medium potencies in bringing about a cure. This is because the astral body's action is, after all, dependent on the middle realm of the human organism.

Now, diphtheria-type symptoms are especially able to give us what we might call intimate insights into the human organism. And these symptoms, manifesting as diptheria-type conditions, should be studied more carefully in relation to the search for methods of healing. There is still a view today, I believe, arising from a more materialistic outlook, that diphtheria should if possible be treated locally—that this condition should be tackled at the local site where it manifests. Naturally numerous other views also dispute this.

The important thing about the development of diphtheria and everything related to it requires further elaboration here since, in the last course,[17] we were not yet able to fully examine this reciprocal action between the four levels of the human organism described by spiritual science. In a different context I suggested that the child's acquisition of speech is accompanied by many kinds of organic processes. The child learns to talk and, while he does so, and while therefore something particular occurs in his respiratory organism, something of a polar opposite nature at the same time occurs in his circulatory organism, the latter of course integrating metabolic processes into itself.

Now, in a quite different context I pointed out that the reciprocal relationship with our surroundings that appears at puberty unfolds inwardly when the child is learning to speak; and that in other words what occurs when the astral body pushes outwards from within at puberty occurs from below upwards in the astralizing process. Learning to talk is, after all, a capacity that develops from below upwards. Thus an astralizing process is involved there too; and we will see clearly how, if we draw the boundary of the respiratory system and circulatory system here (see Fig. 10) a mutual interrelationship occurs between what rises as astralizing process from below upwards (yellow) and the organs that come to meet this astralization from above and intensify their capacity for speech. Our particular interest must focus on what occurs simultaneously here below, for this process down here has the urge to ascend. The whole process is one that rises from below upwards. The whole thing has the urge to rise upwards (arrows, yellow).

If the process that rises from below upwards spreads out too far in an upward direction, and if therefore too strong an upward push of astrality occurs as children learn to talk, this upsurge of astrality represents a disposition to develop diphtheria-type conditions. This is

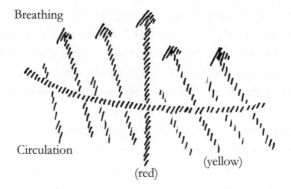

Breathing

Circulation

(red)

(yellow)

Fig. 10

what gives rise to conditions of diphtheria. It is certainly important to give due attention to this.

Now let us also consider the external earth process which has a certain affinity with the process I just described. Let us assume that this is the earth's surface here (see Fig. 11). In a plant which, you can say,

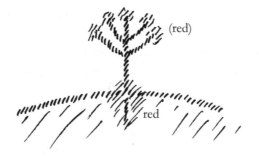

(red)

red

Fig. 11

behaves properly towards the cosmos, the earth participates in the formation of its roots, and this earth influence then diminishes so that the extraterrestrial influences grow ever stronger, unfolding particularly in the flower (red). What unfolds here in the flower is in fact a kind of external astralizing of the flower, which then leads to the development of fruit. If what ought to occur in the normal course of cosmic processes does occur down here (see Fig. 11), it can only engage with water, and we then have what I called the dysentery of the earth. However, what happens when, as I said, the plant develops properly, into a decent plant, always a little way above the surface of the soil where the flower unfolds, can also develop right at the surface of the soil itself (see Fig. 11, bottom red), and then we get mushrooms and fungi. That's how mushrooms grow.

You will likely be close to saying, now, that if mushrooms and fungi develop through this kind of idiosyncratic astralization, then the same process—and this is indeed the case—must occur from below upwards towards the head, as in diphtheria, when this singular astralization process takes place within us. And this is why the tendency to a fungal condition exists in diphtheria. We must be very much aware of this fungal tendency, and take full account of it. A really very hidden process occurs here—all its external aspects are in fact only a sign that irregular astral streams prevail within a person—and this can show us that a school of pathology which concerns itself merely with outer symptoms can of course only gain access to an external manifestation of the whole process. Diphtheria is regarded as a local disorder because only the external symptoms are recognized, without attention to what pushes its way out from within in such a condition. The very sceptical stance people have towards this process can easily be explained if we go back to consider the things that have just been described.

The risk of infection is actually great in diphtheria-related disorders, but why? It is because they develop in direct connection with learning to speak, and occur therefore most widely in children aged between two and four. After this age children are less susceptible. But every process in the human organism that arises in the normal course of things at any particular period can also arise abnormally. This process, therefore, that is really simply a natural process of childhood development can also occur at a later age, albeit in a somewhat modified form, a metamorphosis. When diphtheria occurs at a later age this is in a sense an infantile condition that works on in a person. And the fundamental nature of infancy as you know—in mundane accounts of spiritual-scientific facts we usually need to speak in more psychological terms—is imitation. From an external viewpoint, childhood and infancy certainly involve a process of imitation. And imitation is sought. The organism itself is induced to become imitative when it contracts diphtheria. This is why infection is caused, really, by an urge to become imitative, and such imitation is informed by a subtle sensibility, which we can certainly observe. If we study the matter through spiritual science, we find that the I does, in fact, play a certain role in the process of diphtheria infection. And therefore what develops as fungal infection, the parasitic nature of diphtheria, is more infectious in this condition than in other diseases because the human organism comes to meet it with its imitative urge. As soon as this organism—to put it in a rough and ready way— perceives the diphtheria toxin anywhere, it makes itself receptive to it, relates to it imitatively. For this reason, at an initial stage of the disease, addressing the psyche, strengthening a person through psychological encouragement, will always have a beneficial effect.

With such processes, however, that act so strongly on the organism, we will naturally achieve much less by these means than if we try to discover what I will call the specific antidote to the process occurring there. Here at least I am unaware whether people have made any efforts, even empirically, to discover an antidote to diphtheria-related disorders.[18] One should look for it, for example, in cinnabar up to a medium potency. Cinnabar is the substance whose effects will counteract all the kinds of disorder I have been speaking of. In its very appearance, cinnabar expresses this counteractive capacity. However, an outward appearance only tells us something if we observe it with inner vision. The old doctrine of signatures—which has vanished today simply because people no longer have the necessary powers of observation—relied on instinctive inner vision. It is important however to be able to perceive the inner activity which, basically, is apparent in all external appearances in the world. Someone, therefore, who does not get stuck in a mystic realm, veiling things in all sorts of mystification, but instead retains his healthy common sense, will have to say that vermilion, red cinnabar, is something that in a sense expresses an activity that counteracts fungal processes. Whatever tends towards a colourless state can become fungal. Whereas too strong an astralization of the earth's surface is implicated in fungal growth, in cinnabar-related substances we find a reactivity to this astralization, a counteraction, and therefore the red colour. Wherever reddishness appears in natural processes, astralization is strongly counteracted. To couch this in moral terms, one could say that by reddening the rose tries to defend itself against astralization. Such realms therefore involve an interrelated view

of pathology and therapy that can lead us into this remarkable
relationship of I and astral body to the other organs, in which they grasp
hold of organs or withdraw from them; or manifest excess astral activity
in streams rising from below upwards.

In this way we can gradually come to insight into the whole
human body. We can penetrate and understand it if we pass from
such considerations to something else. And here you will have to consider in turn things I presented last year, but which I will now add to
and extend.

It is very remarkable that the human I—if we now regard its spiritual, psychological, organic and also mineralizing action in the human
being—is a kind of phosphorus bearer. The I elaborates its business of
phosphorus bearing by pursuing this activity to the periphery of the
human being. To bear phosphorus through the human organism,
permeating us with phosphorus, is an I activity. The I carries out this
phosphorus bearing to the outermost limits and periphery of the human
organism in an extraordinarily skilful way. Up to a certain limit, which
it is necessary to adhere to, the I can in fact only bear phosphorus
through the organism by attaching it to other substances and forming
chemical compounds with them. In bearing phosphorus through the
organism, the I basically prevents the chemical release of phosphorus.
Preventing the chemical release of phosphorus is one of the tasks of the
I, except for traces of phosphorus that are in fact necessary if what ought
to be instigated were instigated to a greater degree—if the I proved
unable to stop phosphorus introduced into the organism from being
released. If the phosphorus in us were released, causing an intense effect
on the human organism, a very distinct process would be unleashed.
During these lectures I said that when we are born, thus embodying
physically what previously existed as soul and spirit, images of the
etheric body, the astral body and the I are first engendered. And I said
that everything that is an image of the I really lies in dynamic systems,
movement systems that come into balance. Now this is something we
must be thoroughly aware of at this stage in our reflections. In developing states of balance from imbalance, from upset states of balance—
and whenever I walk or stride I disrupt my balance and have to re-
establish it, and the same thing also occurs through inner processes—

the I needs phosphorus to work in this way. This work is largely carried out through phosphorus.

If the I does not work in such a way as to exhaust its phosphorizing activity in making human dynamics static then, with phosphorus, it approaches what is already an intrinsic image of the I—bringing dynamic movement to stasis in this way. I have spoken of how we need to consider the human being as an aqueous, gaseous and warmth being. Imagine now that you are concerned with the fluid human being and with what enters into the etheric body from the reflected image of the I and the astral body, in which the I is in turn imprinted: here you can see that in this etheric body too it is necessary for a dynamic element, a lack of equilibrium, to continually pass over into balance.

The effects we are considering here are really very subtle.

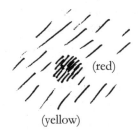

(red)

(yellow)

Fig. 12

And these subtle effects are regulated by virtue of the fact that the human body contains what you might call little free-floating globules or spherules that are, however, in turn connected with the organism's whole movement, also its inner motion. These are the blood globules. What the I does must impact on these globules as it plays into our mobility, also for example into the inner mobility of warmth. These blood globules or corpuscles are thus not globules but are such that their very form reveals how they are geared to leading movements into balance.

It's like this. What the I does when it engages with the human organism's movement capacity meets a boundary in the blood globules and must be halted there. The most intimate reciprocal action must occur there between the human I and the whole human organism. And now what I would call a deeply concealed battle takes place between the ongoing phosphorization of the human being and what lies in the configuring blood process. You see, if phosphorus is taken into the organism in its free state, the blood corpuscles are destroyed by this phosphorizing process. This can lead us to a picture of the remarkable reciprocal action of the I, which is spiritual in nature, spiritual through and through, but which, through the blood corpuscles, is in continual mutual interaction with a physical aspect. In this respect blood is also a 'very special fluid'[19]—an old saying that can be traced back to before Goethe's time. Blood is indeed a very special fluid for it is where the human being's external physical nature enters into reciprocal interplay with the most spiritual aspect we initially bear within us, the I. And when the I enters into this mutual interplay in the wrong way, it is here too that the most ruinous effects can become apparent. If this mutual interplay occurs in the wrong way, a great deal can be destroyed at the physical level, so that we see epithelial disintegration, fatty degeneration of tissue right into muscle fibres, especially striated muscle fibres—since these are where the I is particularly active—and dissolution of the blood corpuscles, etc. This process of disintegration can even make its way right into the bones if there is a disorder of phosphorus processes.

This is clearly apparent in this reciprocal action between the I, which of course involves the astral body too, and the physical body, which draws the etheric body after it. It is very apparent how a continual search for both normality and abnormality occurs, for a normalization advancing to a certain culmination, and how an ebbing then occurs; and how this manifests if, for example, we meet a condition of phosphorus poisoning. In phosphorus poisoning we can observe that initially both the astral body and the etheric body resist what asserts itself both in the physical body and in the I. They resist it with all their power, with the strongest energy the etheric body can muster. The latter tries to make headway against what develops as excessive influence in the I, tries to make headway against it and strengthens its own forces. This is why, at the first stage of phosphorus poisoning, the process so closely resembles another in which, after death, we experience a panoramic review of our life. As you know, this can last for several days—a day and a half, two days, or three. In this review the etheric body is held within the astral body, and we can say that they adhere to each other. They also do this, initially, in the human body when phosphorus poisoning occurs. Everything is developed that can be developed through the collaborative action of astral body and etheric body, and which then likewise occurs in the etheric body's panoramic review after death. In the first stages of phosphorus poisoning therefore, this expended energy will lead to an improvement in the same length of time that such a review would last, followed by a flagging and ebbing of strength. Then, after this ebbing of strength, the abnormal action of the I reasserts itself even more strongly. It is really extraordinarily difficult to combat a real case of phosphorus poisoning. This could only be attempted through vigorous efforts to induce strong collaboration between the astral and etheric—which might be achieved, for instance, by application of powerful blistering plasters to various places on the body. This would no doubt have a beneficial effect. In such a case we have to be clear how far we must go, and develop a feeling for this.

So you see that the physical organism, when the I acts within it, is most strongly engaged by all that one can call the phosphorizing process within us. But when the I intervenes strongly in the physical organism, and thus in a destructive way, the polar opposite must also inevitably occur; and then there is likewise a deficiency of what the I would normally initiate by not taking too strong a hold. In conditions of excessive phosphorus activity, therefore, you will have states of sleeplessness which are simply due to the fact that astral body and I are working their way in and grasping hold too strongly. You can gather this from all that I have said:[20] there will be headaches, delirious states and narcolepsy. In phosphorus poisoning, these and also—prior to general paralysis—anaemic conditions all naturally occur in consequence of what I have described as the reciprocal action between the I and the blood. And then, as a middle ground of these factors, and occurring therefore when the pendulum of the process swings back as it were from what we can call an attack on the blood corpuscles by the I, jaundice-type symptoms appear. And in conditions of jaundice we must certainly see an interplay between psychological and physical factors.

From what I have said here you will see that the process at work in the human being largely involves the I and the astral body working with the forces of the external world within the space encompassed by our skin. They work inwards upon us, and we have to be able to properly discern how their penetration can be regulated; how, in a sense, we can develop a kind of mastery over this penetrating, infiltrating activity.

On a fairly mundane level, based on this view, certain dietary rules emerge by themselves if we know that the excessive action of the I results in irregularities in the stomach, but at the same time in over-vitalization manifesting as abnormal diarrhoea and suchlike. It is necessary, of course, to combat such conditions through diet. The intrinsic I process and that of the astral body within us embody a kind of analysing activity, a breaking down and sundering of what is present as a whole in the outer world. While we have what I would call a primary synthesizing process in the physical and etheric substrata of the human organism, we have analysing processes in the activity of I and astral body; and this analysing activity certainly belongs to the normal processes within us, and comes to such strong, idiosyncratic expression that at an appropriate point this analysing process must also come to a stop. If the I becomes too strong an analyser in relation to phosphates, it analyses them as far as phosphorus-type activity, and then the analysis starts to cause havoc in the human organism. The point where analysis may legitimately act most strongly is, as I showed in last year's lectures, where the analysing process carries through into iron.

This analysing into iron is connected with the blood's iron levels and is in many respects the polar opposite of the analysing process for other metals, which must always in a sense be brought to a halt.

Today, therefore, I wanted to show you how outer phenomena actually provide us with pictures of what emerges from an inner, spiritual realm. An external view of states of health and sickness must be augmented by what we can also know about the inner, spiritual reality within the human being.

On this basis we can gain insights into our medicines and also develop the right basis for answering various questions that have been posed. As far as this is possible, we will discuss all this in the three lectures that still remain.

LECTURE 6

DORNACH, 16 APRIL 1921

YESTERDAY I said that we would direct our thoughts to elucidating the nature of the medicines we have proposed here, and that for this purpose we would try to shape the whole context of these observations. First, though, I would like to note something that may point you to various methodological aspects.

Very often, through imaginative observation of a particular pathology or any general syndrome, we can acquire direct, intuitive knowledge of the respective medicine, and then, as is quite natural, we may be tempted to reflect on this by drawing on prior judgements available to us as external scientific knowledge. In doing so we will find that this is mistaken—that we can't do it like that. This is a very common circumstance which anyone who can undertake esoteric research of any kind—not just in relation to therapy—will come upon frequently. Only by careful pondering, by tracing these things further, do we then find how correct our findings may be. What emerges in research drawing on the imaginative faculty, followed by use of intuition, will always be the correct finding—as long as it is based of course on good powers of cognition. But our judging capacity must always as it were find the right momentum, swing itself up to what we perceive in this way. Here we do have to familiarize ourselves with the extremely complex nature of this human organism, which a rational overview finds the greatest conceivable difficulties in grasping—especially when trying to relate this human organism to the external world once again. This strikes us particularly if we take a somewhat more rigorous view of a circumstance

I mentioned in these lectures: the function of nitrogen in the human organism. As we saw, there is more nitrogen in exhaled than in inhaled air. And materialistic thinking can really only deal with this by saying that the difference is of no significance. This is because a materialistic view of the human being basically cannot show what the function of nitrogen is at all. This only dawns on us if we consider the following.

You know of course that there are all kinds of different theories of nutrition, and that, in interpreting their findings, researchers take up diametrically opposed positions as to the real function in the human organism of protein ingested in food. Why does the human organism need protein? When addressing this problem, I would say that scientists adopt diametrically opposite points of view: some say that the whole structure of human protein organisms is constant, that therefore something constant or relatively so exists here, and that ingested protein undergoes rapid breakdown and really has little significance for the synthesizing, formative capacities of the protein in the human organism. Others by contrast assert something regarded as rather outmoded today—that the protein in us is continually broken down and continually recomposed from the ingested protein. Neither of these two theories, which surface in the most diverse forms, and which represent a kind of diametric opposition, are a true picture of what actually occurs. This is because they both regard protein simply as protein without taking account of the whole human organism.

In this human organism we find a contrast, firstly, between head development—thus the development of nerves and senses—and development arising from the system of limbs and metabolism. There is a diametric contrast here in human nature which it is vital to consider. The graduated structure of the human being, so important for therapeutic considerations, cannot be understood at all without taking this into account. For instance, we certainly won't be able to understand how the lungs behave in the whole human organism without starting from the following research question. In relation to the head organism, certain forces are doubtless predominant. Then we have the chest organism, containing the lungs. The lungs are organs which likewise bear the head forces within them, though more weakly, less intensively, since the same forces pervade the entire human organism in the most varied intensities. And if we now investigate how the I, astral body, and etheric body work on the whole plastic forming and also unforming of the organs, we find, paradoxically, that what forms the lungs is a less intensive version of what forms the head, that the lungs are a meta-morphosis of the head configuration but have just remained behind at an earlier stage. The head progresses further in respect of these same formative forces present in the lungs, which stay behind at an earlier level.

The lungs are a metamorphosis of the head configuration and, by virtue of being an earlier metamorphosis of the head, are suited to their breathing functions. If however the same forces that have remained at an earlier stage in the lungs, and suit it for respiration, advance so that the lungs grow ever more headlike, then they begin to absorb thought forces, the organic powers of thought. In other words, they seek to become an organ of thinking. By trying to do this, by trying too strongly to absorb the forces rightfully located in the head, they acquire a tendency to develop tuberculosis.

We can only understand tuberculosis in the context of the whole human being. We have to see it as indicative of breathing's aspiration to start thinking. The breathing is in fact metamorphosed in the head, and all thinking functions through to the assimilation of perceptions are nothing other than breathing configured in an upward, forward-evolving direction. The head is a more advanced breathing organ which has progressed beyond the scope of the lungs. It simply holds back breathing and, in place of air intake through breathing, replaces it with intake of etheric forces through the senses. Sensory perception is nothing other than a refined breathing process—that is, one taken into the etheric realm. The head breathes and the lungs breathe. But something else—the liver—also breathes in us at a still lower level of this meta-morphic development. The liver is an incomplete lung, an incomplete head form, and also breathes. Here, though, the polar metamorphosis to sensory activity predominates: the absorption and assimilation of nutrients. This is why the development of lungs and liver development occupies a middle position between stomach development on the one hand, and brain and head development on the other.

If you take these ideas as your foundation, you will soon come close to seeing the human organs, certain human organs as such, as basically respiratory organs. All the human organs configured like the brain, lungs and liver are at the same time organs of respiration. As respiratory organs, however, they have the urge to breathe into their surroundings. They therefore excrete carbon dioxide. This excretion of carbon dioxide is the chief aspect of breathing. They absorb oxygen, and this absorption of oxygen and expelling of carbon dioxide is something not only the lung does but is also true of the whole organism, of every organ. It is largely an activity of the astral body, which unfolds its dynamic in sympathy and antipathy. Sympathy corresponds to the capacity of inhalation, while antipathy corresponds to the astral body's capacity to exhale. In my book *Theosophy* you can find a description of the astral body as permeated by forces of antipathy and sympathy. The astral body works in respiration, as antipathy and sympathy, throughout the human being, and we must regard this as the astral body's inner activity.

And here we come to the final point of these observations which tells us that the proteins generally present in us, inasmuch as they belong to organs such as those described, are predisposed to respiration, and come to outward expression through breathing. Yet everything that comes to outward expression also expresses itself inwardly. Let me draw this schematically: a protein-containing organ in you belonging to this organic group I have described expresses itself outwardly by developing respiratory activity (see Fig. 13, red). But by breathing outwardly, [See also Plate 5] it develops another, inner activity, polar opposite to breathing: that of spirit release, of soul release. A soul-releasing activity. By breathing outwards, developing breathing in an outward direction,

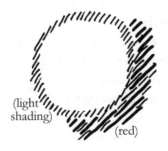

(light shading)

(red)

Fig. 13

you develop an inward activity in soul and spirit, which of course needs no space to unfold. On the contrary, you could say it continually vanishes into space, disappearing from three-dimensional space. But this activity manifests inwardly, in an inward direction, and it is largely due to the property of human protein that it does so. What functions as inner activity in the head is introduced through the senses from without. This is why the head organs contain least spirit. They absorb the spirit from the external world by acquiring it through the senses. The head is the human being's least spiritual organ.

By contrast, human spirituality—specifically initiated in the body in the development of spirit within, of real not abstract spirit—starts in the lung system and works from without inwards, in a contrary direction to breathing. And the most spiritual organs are those belonging to the liver system. They develop the greatest spiritual activity in an inward direction. This can also tell us why head-focused people become materialistic. Since the head can only assimilate external spirituality, they are misled into believing that everything of a mental or spiritual nature is absorbed from the external sensory world. A full-blown intellectual will therefore always also be a materialist. The more of a thinker one is—a head thinker—the more one will tend to become a materialist. If we wrestle our way through to insight with our whole being, on the other hand, starting to become aware of how we think as a totality, with organs lying further back, then materialism ceases to find affirmation in our consciousness.

The activity which comes to expression in breathing is also apparent externally, in the elimination of carbon as carbon dioxide. But the accompanying activity of spiritualization, which unfolds in an inward direction, is connected with nitrogen. Once the nitrogen is expended, it is expelled, you see, for the purpose of spiritualization. The degree to which nitrogen is expelled is a measure of how much our organs are working inwardly towards spiritualization. From this you can gather that someone who does not credit the existence of spirituality will inevitably remain in the dark about the uptake of nitrogen in the human organism. Only once we know that both an inward- and outward-directed activity unfolds every time protein is formed or configured can we understand the role of nutrition. If you examine this process, which is fundamentally a process of respiration with its polar contrasts, you can see that nutrition and digestion border everywhere on processes of respiration. Wherever nutrition and digestion are at work, breathing and spiritualizing processes come towards them. In this spiritualizing process—thus in the other aspect of breathing—we find shaping and modelling forces at work in protein formation, everything that gives us form. And then you can also understand the following: this activity also very much indicates a reciprocal interplay of the astral body and the ether body. The astral body works in our breathing through sympathy and antipathy while the etheric body's activity comes up against the astral body's sympathies and antipathies. Everywhere in the human organism, the ether body and its activities encounter respiration. The ether's actions engage in us predominantly in our fluid parts. We are at least two-thirds water of course. In this aqueous organism, where the etheric body is primarily active, the ether forces manifest physically. In the other organism, a gaseous one, implanted into us from the atmosphere, the forces of respiration come to expression. And so we can also regard what occurs between astral body and etheric body as a reciprocal interplay between water forces and air forces. This interplay of water and air forces continually takes place in us. Neither, of course, is entirely suppressed by the other. This is why we always inhale traces of water vapour with the air, so that ether quality also crosses over into the breathing aspect. Likewise respiratory activity crosses over into intrinsic organs of digestion and nutrition. In so far as they are also formed of protein, they too breathe. You see, one aspect always crosses over into the other, so that one or the other activity always predominates in any particular organ. We can never describe these things in a one-sided way. If we regard a particular organ, say the lungs, as dedicated solely to respiration, we are mistaken. The other activity is always also present, although to a lesser extent. Nutrition primarily occurs through an activity developing in etheric fluidity and physical solidity. In other words, the primary aspect of nutritional and digestive activity is accomplished in a fluid etheric and solid physical realm, while the primary aspect of breathing activity occurs in the gaseous realm, and the primary aspect of I activity, intrinsically spiritual activity, unfolds in diverse states of temperature in relationship of course with this same I.

In the physical organism, spiritual activity embodies an interaction of the I with states of temperature, with all those systems where warmth can work into the physical body. The I must always be allied with warmth, and its activity always proceeds from warmth. If we put a patient to bed and cover him with a blanket, this means nothing other than inviting the I to make suitable use of the increase in warmth thus achieved.

At the same time this highlights human nutrition in general. This is an interaction between tissue fluids, the aqueous domain, in which nutrition and elimination primarily occur, and our actual protein organism. The latter remains relatively stable or constant, only fluctuating as we grow and then becoming more stable and at most undergoing a kind of depletion in the second half of life. In tissue fluid a continual absorption and breakdown of the protein contained in food occurs. And in this activity lie the attacks carried out on what seeks to remain a stable factor in protein synthesis: the internal protein organs themselves. They wish to remain stable, because they seek to inwardly secrete or release soul-spiritual activity. What is accomplished in the process of nutrition is really based on this constant interaction between lively uptake and destruction of proteins and the play of forces that is seeking rest, an extraordinarily dynamic interplay in the protein within us. It is therefore partly a superstition—though it also contains some truth—to say we are built up from the food we ingest. It is superstition because the constructive forces are already present in us through the very fact of being human, are contained in our proteins; and because, on the other hand, we unfold an activity from the other pole that is really an ongoing attack on the stability of our own protein configuration. And so it is not true to say that intake of nutrients sustains human life. It simply isn't true, for it is equally true to say that life is sustained by ensuring the living interplay of forces in tissue fluid. If, therefore, you prepare dishes that stimulate this activity in tissue fluid, then you are sustaining life. You are not doing so, however, by administering nutrients to the body but instead by exerting an impact on the stable forces of the body's proteins. The process you stimulate through intake of food embodies the most primary factor in sustaining life, so that here too we must focus on the process. For instance, substances we know to be very beneficial in children may well have no effect in adults. This is because the child is involved in formative growth and weight increase, and therefore needs intake of substances, needs these to enter him and unfold their forces inwardly. If a particular substance has a good effect in a child, this does not by any means signify that it will work in an adult in the same way. In an adult it may well be far more important simply to sustain the repose-seeking forces in his tissue fluid by activating an appropriate stimulus. If we now turn from everything that develops in the backwards-oriented human organs, in the lungs and liver—the head is of course also backwards-oriented—to consider organs that are more embedded in tissue fluid, in this activity, then we come to the heart enclosed by the lungs as archetype of these. This human heart is formed entirely out of the activity of tissue fluid, and its activity is nothing other than a reflection of the inner activity of tissue fluid.

The heart is not a pump, as I have often remarked, but is more what I would call an instrument for reading or monitoring the activity of tissue fluid. The pumping actions of the heart do not cause blood circulation, but the circulation, rather, gives the heart its impetus. The heart has as little to do with the circulatory function in us as the thermometer has to do with producing external heat or cold. Just as a thermometer is nothing other than an instrument for recording heat and cold, so the heart is an instrument for recording our circulation and what flows into it from the blood's metabolic system. Here we have a golden rule we must faithfully observe if we wish to understand the human being. The modern scientific belief that the heart is a pump that drives blood through the blood vessels is the opposite of the truth. Those who subscribe to the heart-as-pump belief should, if they wish to be consistent, also declare their faith in the capacity of a thermometer to raise the temperature in a room! These two things are really one and the same.

So you see the consequences of an outlook that ignores by far the most important aspect of the human being—the spirit and soul. It overlooks the motion-impelling, dynamic force in us and instead bases everything on mere substance. This outlook seeks to derive from matter the forces which are really impressed upon it. It tries to impose on the heart capacities which in fact it only acquires through the dynamic play of forces informing it.

And so we can say that the opposite of respiration and the release of spirit in us is embodied, in the most advanced and highly organized form, in heart activity and the organ of the heart. Here we find what can be called the polar metamorphosis to mere reconfiguration. If we examine the head, lung and liver we find various stages of reconfiguring metamorphosis. But as soon as we consider the heart in relation to the lungs, we have to speak of a polar metamorphosis, in other words of the fact that the form of the heart is polar opposite to the lungs. And all the organs which develop in a more anterior position, including in most exemplary form the female uterus, are in turn reconfigured stages of cardiac development. I refer to the female uterus since there is also a male uterus, but this is only present as ether body in the man. The uterus is nothing other than a reconfigured heart. This approach is the starting point for developing insight into the human organization.

Now the fats and carbohydrates are what engage with this other activity, which you can say has its centre or comes to rest in the motions of the heart. This is where these fats and carbohydrates exert their action. Of course this extends over the whole body, for just as the whole body breathes and develops spirit, so on the other hand it also deposits substance and elaborates functional systems of forces geared to combustion. This can cast a certain light—and at the same time illustrate how we always pass from true inner observation of the human organism to therapeutic considerations—on the condition that used to be called 'consumption' and has only acquired other names based on theoretical thinking. The condition involves the fact that diverse influences contributing to this disorder, all basically the same in nature, divert the human being from a cosmic sphere and push him towards the earthly— to life in poor dwellings and so forth. All the accounts we have relating to consumption or tuberculosis can be summed up as symptomatic of the fact that people are diverted away from the sun and the cosmos and impelled to lead a life that separates them from sun and cosmos. Thus they lose their joy in cosmic influences, consisting largely in absorption and perception via the senses. In such a person this joy is dulled so that his soul, his whole sensibility, may not permeate the senses, and in consequence descends into the lungs which then seek to become an organ of thinking—to become head—so that their outer form also clearly shows this tendency. The form assumed by the lungs in this disorder shows us that the forces which ossify the human head are coming to expression there, giving rise to indurations of the lung and suchlike. What must we do therefore if we wish to counteract this condition?

To combat the lungs' tendency to become head, we must consider, first and foremost, that this points to a slackening of the necessary astral activity, and to excessive I activity. In other words, I activity starts to overcome astral activity. This must be remedied. All external sensory impressions stimulate I activity in particular. And assimilation of sensory stimulus continues its way inward throughout the human organism and culminates in salt deposits. These deposits are not properly regulated in someone with a tendency to consumption. We must therefore offer support here and try to counteract what the lungs are no longer capable of by administering highly concentrated external applications of salt. Salt rubs, applied externally, will counteract the processes of induration that develop from within outwards.

Externally applied salt rubs must naturally also be enhanced in their effect by efforts to induce the inner organism to absorb and accept what is trying to enter from without. One can also prescribe salt baths, highly concentrated salt baths, but one still has to induce the organism to really engage with this inwardly, or in other words respond to it from within. Here you can weigh up the following, which partly follows from what we discussed last year.

To stimulate the organism to develop from within an activity that responds to and regulates certain external organizing forces, we need to administer small doses—tending towards homoeopathic dilutions—of mercury. In this respect mercury is an important medicine, an important regulator. General dosage guidelines will be particularly applicable here. To sum up what I have said previously, the system of metabolism and limbs is the one that most closely resembles external nature. If this system lacks something, and we need to intervene here, we have to use the low potencies. As soon as we come to the middle system, medium potencies are needed. And when we wish to work from the head, or as soon as we wish to work from what is connected with the activity of the spirit in the head, we need the higher potencies. In this case, since we are

concerned with the activity of the lungs, this is part of our middle
system, and the mercury potency must be a medium one. Wherever we
count particularly on a medicine that works on the head organization,
and from there back through the whole organism, the highest potencies
are required, and these will be especially beneficial wherever we decide
that silicon compounds are called for. By their very nature silicon
compounds require the highest dilution because they always gravitate
towards the head and the body's periphery—which also belongs to the
head system. In calcium compounds, on the other hand, when use of
these is called for due to other reasons, we will almost invariably be right
to stop short of the highest potencies and instead use the low potencies.
To sum up, a rule of thumb for potentizing is whether we need to
intervene in the system of limbs and metabolism, the middle rhythmic
organization or the head organism. In the latter case, though, we must
of course also remember that the head organism in turn sends strength
through the whole organism from the other direction. One can for
example discover that a foot complaint is really a head disorder in
disguise and originates in the head. Then we should not try to cure it by
addressing the metabolism, but rather the head. Here we can use high
potencies of a substance which might be good in low potencies if it were
a matter of inducing a curative effect originating in the metabolism.
These things all certainly have a rationale, which must gradually be
discovered. We will only proceed properly here if we engage in careful
and precise observations of the outcome of our research. But the ways
we should proceed must be sought as outlined here.

It is also important to remember that no one is entitled to speak
about specific cures unless he really carefully compiles and remembers
what his experiences have taught him, for every single such experience is
of course also instructive and bears fruit for subsequent cases. Now if
you take account of what I have said here, you will find that it no longer
seems nearly so mysterious if a disorder affects both brain and liver
simultaneously. The liver is just a metamorphosed brain. If we find
simultaneous liver degeneration and deterioration of the brain ganglia,
these two conditions lie in precisely the same direction. Here we find, in
fact, a form of disease intensified in comparison to what causes tuberculosis. It is merely an intensified metamorphosis of tuberculosis. In this

case, therefore, we need to administer mercury in a less dilute form and, as external application, rather than external applications and baths using ordinary sodium salt, common salt, we will need to resort to calcium salts.

You will gather that possible sources of error lie in wait everywhere, and that we can really only discover the right course of action by observing the human organism from within outwards. Someone, for instance, might easily come along and say that a particular disorder can be cured with mercury. And this treatment will achieve some effect or other. But the disorder in question is by no means inevitably connected with syphilis, and if the person in question imagines that anything cured with mercury must be connected with syphilis he may well be mistaken. In the same way you will now understand the things a bit better which I said when talking about 'mental disorders' last year. When I spoke of softening of the brain several days ago, I was of course referring to paralytic disorders. But the term 'paralysis' is somewhat vague. There is always a sense that one is referring to an externally manifesting syndrome. But now, of course, we have to ask what I meant by saying, last year, that the real causes of psychological disorders must be sought in organ deformities. This is indeed true, and is true to such a degree that considering symptoms of mental disorder alone will not lead to any useful outcome—nothing much will result. One can actually say that very similar psychological complexes can be traced back to very different causes. In so-called 'mentally ill' patients, we always need to look for an organ deformity, some organ or other that is not functioning properly; and then we must ask why it isn't functioning. We will find it is because forces of stable protein synthesis—not the variable but the stable forces—have become defective. So there is something in the patient that continually seeks to destroy the original shape and structure of a particular organ. And for this reason it does no good to focus too much on what is happening in the tissue fluids and, of course, represents the other pole of metabolism. Thus in starting from the symptoms we won't get anywhere with what intrinsically belongs to metabolism. On the other hand it will be extraordinarily important to seek insight into mental illnesses in eliminated substances. This will give us important reference points. It is extremely important to study the nature of eliminations in someone with mental illness. Last year I said that certain types of mental illness present as a compulsion to form imaginations and inspirations, and this is indeed what inner release of spirit signifies.

If this kind of compulsion is present, this is basically because the organ has become damaged. If the organ is not defective but normally constituted, it does indeed develop imaginative capacity but this remains unconscious. Once it has been damaged it is no longer able to develop imagination properly. On the one hand the organ is defective and in consequence a compulsion to develop imagination arises, and on the other the imagination remains unsecured by the organ and therefore appears as hallucination and so forth. We can see it like this: if we have an organ and the imaginations developing within it (see Fig. 14, below, red) which then radiate into the rest of the human organism (Fig. 14, light shading) and are perceived, then if the organ is deformed the developing imagination (red) cannot unfold properly in its plasticity and thus, being abnormal, it impresses itself on conscious awareness.

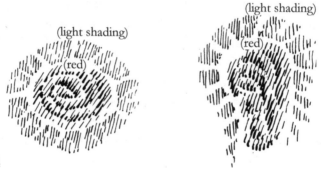

Fig. 14

Then we find the patient has hallucinations and visions. On the other hand, the organ is not functioning properly, and this gives rise to the urgent desire for real imaginations. Such things become clear simply by gaining an insight in this way into their inner nature.

We will end here and listen to Dr Scheidegger's lecture.[21] When we reconvene we will address the questions that have been asked and also explain more about our medicines.

LECTURE 7

DORNACH, 17 APRIL 1921

I will turn now to pharmacology, which we will discuss also in relation to medicines we have already tried to develop. Let me note specifically that I have no interest in giving an account of my train of thought in arriving at a potential medicine. My concern instead is for you to understand how a certain substance can be used medicinally. The insight we need into a substance is one I would like to see unfolding in each physician's soul, giving it value as a medicine. Today therefore I would like to use our discussions to probe into ways in which we might come to see that a particular substance could be a medicine. A foundation for this, as I must of course first mention, is familiarity with the major principles of anthroposophical insight into the human being. A proper interpretation of a medicine can only arise if we are, as it were, energized from below to shed an anthroposophical light upon our whole enquiry. You will also see therefore that what I have said in preceding days will flow into our deliberations today.

Let us assume that the plant in particular allows us to study the reciprocal action between our surroundings and ourselves as human beings. By first versing ourselves in processes at work in the plant, we can gain the right view of how mineralization processes work their way through into our interior. If we embark on this kind of enquiry—and this is of course based on everything we have considered in the past few days—we must be clear that in the whole plant development process, the process whereby roots, leaves, blossoms, seeds and so forth are shaped, lies something configured out of the whole cosmos. We must also realize that this process, especially as it takes shape in plant forms—including their inner forms—cannot be replaced by some kind of merely artificial synthesis, in other words by chemical compounds. Only in the very rarest cases can this natural synthesis be replaced by an artificial one. We have to be clear about the following, for instance. Within plant development processes, the root of a plant is more or less bound up with the inner forces of the earth's surface. Now human beings are plantlike in the sense that their soul and spirit grow from above downwards. Our head contains many of the same forces that interact with the forces of the earth itself, and there is a profound affinity between what forms as root in the plant and all the forces at work in the human head. Whenever we seek to understand the process at work in the root parts of a plant, therefore, we will need to see that this process has a reciprocal relationship with the human head. But let us now embark on our enquiries by starting with specific details, so that you can see how such enquiries should be conducted. Let us for instance consider the gentian root, *Gentiana lutea*, and pursue the following train of thought: The gentian is a plant which expresses itself outwardly in strong flowers. In the root, therefore, we will have forces that are drawn strongly towards the floral aspect. In other words, these root forces are somewhat weak. The gentian plant expends itself a great deal in flowers and leaves. Nevertheless, the whole form of the flower shows that the plant's root aspect is still strongly present. Therefore we cannot necessarily count on the gentian having a strong effect on what proceeds directly from the human head organization and is intrinsic to it, that is, as external physical effect, but instead we can expect it to work primarily on the respiration-promoting activity emanating from the head. And since we always find a polar action in the organism, we must imagine that the digestive organs themselves can be induced to breathe more strongly—in the sense described yesterday—if we use the gentian's roots. In other words, we stimulate the stomach and intestines to respire more actively; and must then consider what we have learned during these lectures—that to stimulate this respiratory activity, plant substance must be processed, in this case by making a decoction of the roots. We must use a root decoction. You see, we can really penetrate all this with under-standing. Here we first look at external aspects, discovering that the gentian root has a bitter taste and a strong smell—and so this is something that works very strongly on the astral. We therefore have here an action exerted on the astral nature of our digestive parts. But the gentian root also contains sugar. I have repeatedly pointed out, as you will recall, that when we assimilate sugar in the human organism this process greatly stimulates I activity. You can even confirm this statistically, as I have said, by studying how nations with little I activity such as those in eastern Europe, the Russian peoples, in whom the I is less predominant, have very low national annual sugar consumption, whereas the English, in whom the I develops extremely brisk activity— and this is true in general the further west we go—have a proportionately higher sugar intake, as statistics demonstrate. Such things must certainly be taken account if we wish to develop understanding of the world.

A further characteristic of the gentian root is that it is rich in fatty oils. Fatty oil works strongly on the lower respiration when it passes into the digestion, since it strengthens motility, the inner mobility of stomach and intestines. You can see therefore how one can describe in detail what occurs here within the human organism. Immediately one notices that astral activity is stimulated, thus stimulating respiratory mobility of the stomach and intestine. And then one sees that the intestines develop a brisker activity and that the stomach is strengthened. The whole thing takes effect to create a condition that always arises when the astral body is strengthened: mineralization processes then only occur in us in so far as this consolidates the organs themselves, hence making them stronger. What occurs here is the gentle influence of the I through sugar. So we could say that by using a decoction of the gentian root we induce brisk activity in the astral body, while the root's sugar content enables the I to support this. However, the fact that the I boosts the effect signifies a danger. If the I whips things up from below, a polar reaction arises in turn in the head, and we can find that such patients get headaches as a side effect. Yet what I have described does indeed take effect in all these directions. Basically we have an activating and stimulating of intestinal activity, and we will therefore use such a medicine either on its own or in some combination, whenever we notice that symptoms and signs are related to loss of appetite, dyspepsia for instance, and especially various forms of abdominal congestion. We can also see how this gastric and intestinal activity stimulates metabolism in general, inwardly enlivening and activating it, and by this means we can also counteract tendencies to gout and rheumatism. In the gentian root we will also be drawing on something which combats fever, if only to a mild degree. When intestinal function is undermined, this calls forth a febrile reaction in our upper system. If we strengthen the lower system, therefore, we create a counterweight to our upper pole, and have thus administered something that counteracts fever.

These are the kinds of exploration we need to pursue to arrive at the specific ways in which the external world relates to our inner processes. It is quite correct to state that external influences stream in on us. Rosenbach is an instance of someone who has done excellent preparatory work in this field.[22] But to speak abstractly of influences fails to grasp that what works upon us from without derives from tangible realities. There is a real relationship between the root nature of plants, the forces active in roots, and what these do when they enter us. Things we otherwise only characterize in the abstract as influences can really be grasped by such insights. And spiritual science is concerned to elaborate really specific aspects, the actual processes at work.

With this in mind let us turn to an extraordinarily instructive plant, herb bennet or wood avens—*Geum urbanum*[23]—and once again make use of its root as a decoction. It is extremely interesting to investigate herb bennet while also remembering what we have just said about the gentian root. Once again we must of course assume that using the root will have a reciprocal effect on head forces. In herb bennet root we have a bitter taste, really extremely tart. The root of herb bennet contains essential or volatile oils, and we can therefore easily predict that it will affect parts of the organism that are not within nor as close to the intestinal tract as the parts we spoke of in relation to the gentian root. Here there is more of a connection with what needs to happen earlier, in the stomach or maybe even the oesophagus. The most important constituents to consider in herb bennet root are its starches, the amylum content, so that we appeal in a sense to forces that assimilate more intensively than is necessary for sugar. In assimilating amylum the power of engagement has to be held back more, so that the sugar can first be drawn out. You can see therefore that we really have to trace the processes at work. The herb bennet root also contains a tannin, and we must always consider this when studying the medicinal actions of a substance. A tannin means that the substance in question acts upon whatever the tannin encounters in a way that strongly approaches the physical; and we must therefore locate the whole action of herb bennet root closer to the I than to the astral body. Because I stimulus is enhanced, we have here an activity in the lower part of the human organism as polar effect to stimulation of the head, which the I brings about there. We are concerned here with what I would call outward digestion, an engagement with substances while they are still in the stomach, before they pass on into the intestinal tract. If I may put it like this, the neurosensory apparatus still present in the intestine—for everything is spread out over the whole human organism—is stimulated, and we therefore find I activity predominant here.

What will be the consequence of this? That firstly we have in herb bennet root a strongly anti-pyretic action. Secondly, though, we will be able to work from more anterior digestive processes on more posterior ones, the actual intestinal processes, by not foisting such a burden on the latter. By this means we will be able to combat diarrhoea in particular, or intestinal muco-enteritis, if we consider that these disorders arise when too much is expected of more interior digestive processes. So you see that these enquiries all lead us to insight into how external forces penetrate what lies in the human interior.

Since it is especially important to consider the action of roots, let us take one more root—*Iris germanica*, garden or bearded iris. Here too we make a decoction. The outward appearance of this iris already tells us that it works strongly on the I. Its distasteful smell and bitter taste immediately betray the fact that we have here something in which the I enters into strong physical interplay with the external world. The garden iris root also contains something that greatly stimulates this physical activity—tannic acid. And once again there is amylum here, which stimulates I activity. Finally the iris root also contains something that takes physical effect wherever it appears, when stimulated to do so: we have resins. All this stimulates the I to very brisk activity. And this lively activity of the I, this impelling power of the I, can be detected in increased urine activity and a certain purgative effect. These are the external manifestations of I activity. And the condition we can combat by this means becomes clear simply by asking what the human organism suffers when all this is not in order. We find dropsy and similar disorders; and the iris decoction provides something with which we can try to combat dropsy-type conditions and also dropsy itself.

These are the kinds of consideration to be weighed up. Now, if we rise somewhat higher up the plant we can consider its herbaceous parts. Let us take a characteristic plant such as *Majorana hortensis*, or marjoram. But let's be clear: when we ascend to the stalks and foliage, nature itself now accomplishes certain processes which we ourselves first had to undertake with the roots. If we take the herbaceous parts it is not good to make a decoction since we need its subtler forces—which we can obtain by making an infusion. These forces pass from the leaves into the infusion. And here again you can detect through your senses what is present here. In this infusion of marjoram you have its distinctive taste, which we could call a 'warming taste'. This taste has at the same time a somewhat bitter quality. And then you also have something which clearly testifies to an outward-directed action: the aromatic fragrance due to its essential oils. And in addition there is something needed only to intensify all this to a marked degree, which does not come to physical expression as quickly as the other qualities but does so only on passing through the the stomach and entering intestines. All kinds of salts are contained in the leaves, specifically in marjoram. You can therefore discover—and these things are realities—that this infusion of leaves will act especially on the respiratory activity of the internal organs. It induces a certain respiratory activity in the internal organs. You can see this from the fact that the infusion has a diaphoretic action, causes perspiration—and so in other words stimulates inner respiratory activity in the organs. It causes perspiration, and through this reaction strengthens the internal organs' activity. Administering a marjoram infusion counteracts catarrhal colds; but on the other hand it can also be used to treat uterine weakness.

All these things will come into clearer focus if we now pass to the action of the flower. Let us first observe this action in the plant in nature, where it reveals itself most clearly—for instance wherever many small flowers unfold in an inflorescence, as in the elder, or *Sambucus nigra*. And let us be clear that the forces here shooting into the plant are closely connected with the periphery of the earth and contain cosmic influences and streams. We can see this from the fact that the elder-flower also contains essential oils. But notably it can be discovered in the sulphur content of the elderflowers. Here we have something from the mineral realm that turns out to be especially effective in stimulating respiration, but from the other direction, that of the respiratory organization itself—as opposed to stimulus of respiration in the digestive organs and in what attaches to them before respiration of the actual breathing organs takes hold of them. The elderflower, when used—this is fairly obvious—as an infusion, especially stimulates the human organism's ether activity, and only on a roundabout route through ether activity does it also stimulate the astral body. In other words, respiration in the upper posterior organs is stimulated particularly—but not so much in the head organs as in those that belong to breathing itself. Naturally, reactions arise everywhere here, and these of course show us that, in this instance, discharges and perspiration occur. And now it is the respiratory organs which are stimulated. Otherwise normal respiratory function is given an impetus and—since this inevitably has an effect on the blood too—this in turn stimulates blood circulation from within. From all this we can detect that such a medicine can act against catarrh, can combat perspiration retention, and is useful in cases of hoarseness and coughing. Also, since the direct action that previously arose now appears as polar effect, it can be used in rheumatoid conditions.

You see, it is important always to anticipate the medicinal powers of an agent by considering its mode of action. Now let us consider that it may be necessary to act on the head organization in particular. What is dependent on the head organization?

Digestion is dependent on it, as the head organization's polar counterpart. The head organization governs the coarser aspect of digestion—the cause of so many very severe diseases. We must therefore be clear that we can significantly affect the head from these coarser digestive processes, and that whenever we work on the digestion from within we inevitably also give rise to effects that radiate into the head, and from there unfold their action. We must of course keep an overview of all sorts of diverse aspects, and despite first seeking to give a herbal medicine internally do so in such a way that it affects the head. This can be achieved especially if we use seeds. By their very nature seeds are very well suited to work directly on coarser digestive processes. By doing so, however, and producing reactions, they also affect the head. But it is very difficult to raise a medicinal action from the digestion so that it enters the head. In the case of seeds, therefore, it is good to resort to a decoction once more—in very concentrated form—as long as the patient can tolerate this. We can study this in particular if we look at the medicinal actions of caraway seeds, of a decoction of these seeds. A decoction contains, firstly, essential oils and thus exerts strong effects on the I, and also, again, something with a very strong physical action, wax and also resins, which likewise induce very strong effects in the physical realm. The strength of this action is apparent in the spicy smell. Then, in this decoction, we specifically have galactose.

If you connect all this with our observations in the course so far, it has an extremely strengthening effect on I activity, a substantial effect on the sense and nerve activity hidden in the digestive organs. The effect works particularly on this weak activity of the senses and nerves concealed within the digestive organs and distributed there in a very weakly developed metamorphosis. In relation to our lower organism, a decoction of this kind really works on something that one can call a subconscious metamorphosis of our external sensory perception. You can say that it stimulates our digestive system to perceive the process developing there. And this is why this is such a good medicine for use in enemas. Using it as an enema we invoke a process that inevitably affects the action of the senses and nerves because it administers from without the subtle forces contained in the caraway seeds, and thereby awakens a kind of subconscious perception in the organs of digestion. Sluggish tissue fluid is stimulated in particular. So by invoking a process that strengthens the nerves and senses, perception is strongly transposed into our interior. We start to perceive in our digestive organs, and this counteracts and stands as it were as an opposite pole to what happens when an inner activity of our organism—which can also now be perceived, though largely in inner perception—begins to manifest in eruptive conditions. By perceiving our own organism very strongly when it develops organic activity of this kind, so that in fact we perceive ourselves, we exert a dampening and thus curative effect on such an activity—which is an outward-directed perception from within—by developing an opposing activity of senses and nerves resembling a metamorphosis of external perception. This medicine can be beneficial in treating stomach cramps, colic-type conditions and flatulence.

The following further process is really very interesting to observe. Imagine very vividly the kind of subconscious activity that develops here. This subconscious activity very closely resembles that of external perception but has, in a sense, been transposed into our interior. Consider that external perception and reflex activity have a certain mutual connection: when subconscious perceptions arise they can immediately trigger defensive reactions. So let us consider this interaction between perception and defensive reaction, and now transpose this onto the inner activity of tissue fluid. You carry out this activity of external perception by floating as it were in the air. If I draw this schematically, we can here picture the air around us, permeated by light and so on (see Fig. 15, light shading), [See also Plate 6]

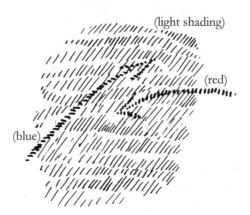

(light shading)

(red)

(blue)

Fig. 15

and here we have external perception (red) unfolding in this direction, the inner response unfolding in this direction (blue). In every sense organ we do indeed have an interplay of external action and inner reaction. If we want to give an outward, abstract picture of this, we should at least not use the one chosen in the modern materialistic view, which states that a centripetal and centrifugal nerve activity is involved here. This interpretation is no cleverer than saying, that when one exerts pressure on a rubber ball it recreates its original shape through a different force than the opposite counter-pressure. It is no cleverer to speak of motor nerves than to explain the elasticity of a ball by saying that after pressing on it one posits some kind of centre to its interior which then pushes out again. What happens in fact is merely that the original shape is re-established. The effect does not require any special nerves since the whole process of action and counteraction is embedded in astrality and I nature.

But now picture this whole process as occurring by a roundabout route through ether activity in the tissue fluid (see Fig. 16, yellow). [See also Plate 6, right]

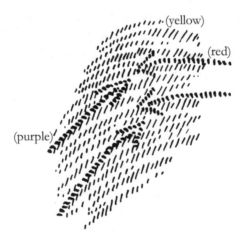

Fig. 16

A sensory process does not of course occur in the tissue fluid under normal circumstances, but it can be induced by what I just described. Then a kind of contracting tendency arises, an approach towards the organism which I wish to indicate here in the same way as action in perception. But this (red) is a process that in a sense storms against the outward-directed force (purple) in the tissue fluid. This asserts itself and this other counteracts it. Thus we transpose a sensory process, a metamorphosis of the sensory process, into tissue fluid. It is extremely interesting to observe how we here transpose a metamorphosis of the external sensory process into tissue fluid. Now we must see where we can find something like this happening in daily life, so that a kind of metamorphosis of the sensory process arises within us, you could say as a concentrated sensory process in tissue fluid. This happens when milk forms and is secreted during female lactation. Here we have a metamorphosis of external sensory processes transposed inwards and concentrated as breast milk. Now let us assume that, when needed, this process of lactation does not adequately occur—then we have very good reason to bring about this concentrated and inwards-transposed sensory process. And in a decoction of caraway seed we have what invokes such a process and promotes lactation.

I have cited these examples to show how we can regard the whole working and activity of this human organism and its interrelationship with what exists in the surrounding world. Consider what I have presented to you here. Consider it in precise detail. In the decoction of the caraway seed there is resin and wax, and therefore something whose consistency invokes especially strong physical effects. Thus the resin, the wax, is extraordinarily similar to my outer sensory impressions, but just inwardly concentrated.

And this seed, again, contains essential oil and galactose, which stimulates the reactivity of the I. Here you have everything present together that also exists in the sensory process: the external stimulus, the inner reaction penetrating as far as the I. Now you metamorphose this sensory process by virtue of the fact that, instead of a sensory perception, you transpose this reciprocal effect inwards, into the system of forces of the tissue fluid. Then you have something that invokes an inner sensory process in you—which is what the process of lactation is. You will see how we can come to understand the whole organism by this means.

These are the enquiries we need to engage in if we wish to gain understanding of the inner action of external substances. If we take the example of mineral or metal medicines we will easily be able to gain insight into something we already learned in relation to the action of a herbal medicine. But we will also be able to see here that something has happened to the mineral whereby mineral qualities have been carried through into the plant process. What occurs in mineralization and vegetabilization involves a reconfiguring of mineral forces. Something in the process of healing therefore depends on the reconfiguration of mineral forces. Let us assume that we establish a clinic, surround it with fields and fertilize these fields with various mineral substances. We now have an active soil and are aware of what it contains, and cultivate diverse plants there for their roots, leaves, fruit and so forth. Thus we control the whole process, which involves the plant transforming minerals into medicines. We can intensify this by growing plants such as those we were just describing, which can indeed be treated in this way. That's what we are trying to do at our institute in Stuttgart,[24] that's how it has to be done. But then we can go still further. The medicine we have obtained in this way through the plant can in turn be used as a kind of fertilizer, which will intensify its action. We will obtain something which renders normal physical trituration substantially more effective—in other words transforms it into something extremely active, by asking nature itself, the forces active in nature, to prepare it for us. We must also then of course be clear about the following. For instance, we can ask how a mineral or metal preparation is to be effective, how it should act. The salts, which by the way are also mineral medicines, engender more of an interior effect. The most peripheral activities, however, are influenced precisely by mineral or metal substances, which one can say are the most inherently consistent. Here we will have to weigh up the best course of action, but always, as I said, drawing on the foundation of spiritual-scientific insights, for otherwise one's thoughts fragment and shoot off down all sorts of mistaken paths. Spiritual-scientific ideas give the proper direction to such thinking. For instance, we can have a particular metal, and know that the interior of the human organism can only engage with it very weakly. So here the activity of the I needs greatly stimulating, for the I is what reaches down as it were into the inner nature of substance, arranges this inner nature according to its purposes and then invokes I activity within the organism. Since the I can be strengthened in this activity by the astral body, if we use metals, use minerals, we must always ensure that we also stimulate I activity or astral activity—which then works back upon the I—or the interaction between astral activity and I activity. We can for example do this as follows. We prepare a metal ointment and apply it. We apply it, let us say, to treat a skin rash. In doing so we activate I activity peripherally. This I activity is likewise stimulated through the person's inner reaction. Within him, initially, intensified nerve and sense activity develops in a particular organ, and from there intensified respiratory activity by passing over into the astral realm. And then we obtain an action, emanating from within, of forces that counteract the skin rash. In this way we call upon the whole body to combat the skin rash.

We can of course generally study the effects of different metals and minerals. In lead, for instance, you have something that exerts an extremely powerful effect on the activity of nerves and senses, and then in turn on associated internal respiration—but also on the internal respiratory activity which occurs for instance in the outer, peripheral organs. So if we use lead when we need to induce an effect as has just been described, we can find it to be very beneficial—used as ointment or also given by mouth. Administered internally we must of course be clear that we are calling forth a reaction in the upper organism by stimulating the activity of the digestive organs. If we use carefully prepared ointments on the upper organism, we are working directly on this upper system itself. And if a patient has some kind of debility in the head, only poorly developed activity of the nerves and senses, and likewise deficient respiration, such lead treatments can achieve a great deal as long as we stop short of a toxic dose. In all such things, construed from what we have learned in recent days and also from our previous course, the following is important to remember.

A very important contrast exists here. Metals that tend more towards silver are in a sense polar to all those which tend towards lead. In relation to these things, of course, our mineral classification systems are really very inadequate indeed. In a system of mineral classification more in accord with nature, such affinities and relationships between metals would have to be considered, and then we would see that lead compounds and lead itself are at one end of the scale while silver is at the other, and aurum, gold, for instance, in the middle. The other metals would all be ranged somewhere along this scale. Silver and lead are polar opposite to each other because silver acts directly on the limbs and metabolism, doing so in a very peripheral way—acting to a large degree on the outward-oriented aspect of the organism of limbs and metabolism. Lead, by contrast, works on the outward-oriented aspect of the head organism. In other words, silver stimulates nerve and sense activity in the system of metabolism and limbs, from there promoting an activity that permeates the whole body and stimulates respiration in all I referred to yesterday as a metamorphosis of the central heart organ.

By contrast, all that issues from lead acts on the nerve and sense activity of the head, and on the activity of breathing stimulated from there. Thus it has a stimulating effect on all that is embodied in the other metamorphosis, the configuration of the head, of the lungs, of the liver, and therefore those organs which in a sense enclose and encompass our other organization in the same way that the lungs encompass the heart. This organization really reveals the archetypal form of what we are in our entirety as circulatory organism. We have the lungs that enclose the heart, so that the breathing system in a sense encompasses and embraces the circulatory system. But we likewise have a broader kind of respiration if we consider the human being in the configuration of brain, lungs and liver, in other words the whole upper, posterior system, and this respiration encompasses all blood vessels together with the heart. The upper, posterior system in this way encloses and encompasses the digestive organization and also the sexual organization. The organization is such that the upper, posterior system in us really encloses the lower, anterior part of us. These two aspects interpenetrate, so that the upper, posterior parts are superimposed upon the lower and anterior parts, and this mutuality chiefly manifests in the reciprocal relationship between heart and lungs. If we carefully observe this and study the rhythmic aspect within this interaction, and then also the activity of nerves and senses above and behind—which naturally has its other pole in the forward and lower system—and if we consider the processes at work in the metabolism and limbs in the anterior and lower parts, and in turn in their other elaboration in the upper and posterior parts, then the whole human being stands before us. And then, accordingly, we can understand the other processes at work in us.

From this point of departure we will proceed tomorrow to a specific discussion of our own medicines, during which some questions that have been raised will find their natural answers.

LECTURE 8

Today's lecture will be a colourful pot pourri of further, wide-ranging comments to extend what has already been said about our medicines. Initially, in a way similar to yesterday's efforts to consider the world of plants, I would like to focus on interpreting mineral-related processes that affect us. The approaches we need here are more complicated since, as soon as we pass to the mineral realm, we no longer have such precise, conclusive parallels as between the defined entities of plant and human being. Instead, the one passes more directly into the other, and distinctions are therefore difficult. When producing medicines—and this is something you must especially consider in relation to our own medicines—it is not merely a matter of using a particular substance but rather of incorporating one process, within whose living context the substance exists, into another. Thus, when the action of a certain medicine becomes known, we must frequently consider how this action induced, in a sense, in one direction, can be checked and curtailed in another. For instance, in relation to the medicine we make with lead and honey, the latter processed in a certain way (as you can find documented) it becomes possible to see how the action of the lead is in a sense meant to be kept in check by the action of honey. The action of lead on all the I-governed developmental processes within us is in fact enormously powerful.

You recall how we described a physical activity within, or rather emanating from the human head, then an etheric impression, an astral impression, an I impression. The I primarily, as we said, impresses itself in the movement system. The action of lead works with particular force on this I impression, in association with the astral impression. Lead's action very much involves an extremely hidden force of nature, and for esoteric observation there is extraordinarily profound significance in witnessing the effects of lead. These effects are of very great importance for our being before it ever embarks on its descent into physical life. It is here that the actions of lead are especially significant. Lead, you see, not only exerts the effects familiar to us, but also, very largely, the polar opposite effects. And these polar opposite effects stream in from the cosmos whereas the effects we are familiar with radiate out into the cosmos from the earth. One could draw a diagram of this as follows: if this is the earth's surface, the familiar actions of lead radiate outwards (drawing, arrow) [See also Plate 7]

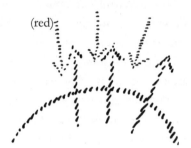

(red)

Fig. 17

whereas the polar opposite actions stream in from all sides. They have no centre from which their radiations emanate, are not centralized forces, but are forces that work in from the periphery (red). These peripheral forces are particularly connected with the development of spirit and soul in us, and their realm is one we must really depart from, largely depart from, when we embark on our descent into the earthly sphere. This is why lead's opposite forces are invoked in the earthly sphere, and why these are then toxic. This is in fact a general, universal secret we should be fully aware of: that everything spatially connected with the human being's soul and spirit nature—which we can therefore generally speak of as a spatial relationship—is toxic within our organism, so that really the very meaning of poison must be derived from this. What we find here, therefore, is a strong spur or stimulus, a kind of whipping up of these I-reflecting forces within human nature. And everything that occurs in cases of lead poisoning primarily tends towards thorough destruction and dehumanization of the human being's form and image, in so far as he is an I. All possible symptoms that signify a gradual transition into bodily non-existence—though of course we die before we reach this point—right down to voice loss and so forth, through to states of unconsciousness and stupor, testify to the fact that our innate developmental forces are being thoroughly destroyed. You see, the principle of human development is destroyed, with the destruction coming from our upper organism, and this upper organism is polar opposite to the lower. Something which is a destructive element in the upper organism in large quantities acts constructively in small quantities, in dilution, from our lower organism.

In passing I would like to say here that, in my view, the never-ending dispute between homoeopathy and allopathy will only be resolved once people can study constituent aspects of the human being as spiritual science describes them. Whereas the principle of homoeopathy cannot be in doubt, or ought not to be at least, given the wealth of empirical findings it offers, those who take the opposite stance and are not in the habit of basing conclusions just on the evidence—for homoeopaths always take a more phenomenalist approach than allopaths, who invariably taint their medical rationale with all sorts of prejudices, all kinds of extraneous deliberations and tendentious views about the human organism—will find it difficult to understand the principle that a substance with a morbid effect in large quantities can have a thera-peutic effect in small ones. This principle does not actually entirely accord with the facts, but only does so if we extend it by saying that what causes a morbid effect in our lower organism exerts a medicinal action in small quantities where its effect proceeds from our upper organism, and vice versa. This reformulation of the homoeopathic principle would be the only suitable way of resolving the dispute.

If we turn back from this little parenthesis to a medicament in which we seek to achieve an effect through a particular way of processing lead and honey, you can see how, from below, we counteract by means of very dilute lead the forces that destroy the human form. This is con-tained in the action of lead. Now we try to build up this I-configuring power in a patient. You see, here we transpose I activity into the physical organism, and by making a person physically well we render him mentally weak in respect of everything that should work up, also organically, from below. On the one hand we bring a person back to his proper course of development, since developmental forces are defective, by using the action of lead in response to certain processes of disease. But weakening which runs parallel with inducing a person to develop his self-configuring powers once again can easily reach a stage where we undermine the forces proceeding from his I and astral body, and particularly those issuing from the I. So we can say that we cure what a person acquired, or rather acquired as a deficiency when he entered earthly life, but we weaken him in relation to what he needs to develop organically while he lives this life. The added action of honey, however, in turn counteracts this, and in other words strengthens the forces issuing from the I. You see, in developing such a medicine, it is largely a matter of understanding what actually happens within us.

Now if we wish to understand the actions of the mineral realm in us, we have to examine how minerals act within the earth. Here we first have to familiarize ourselves with the significance of salts in the earth's evolution. In evolution, the salts signify what the earth accomplishes. What the earth accomplishes is contained in the action of salts. By developing salt, it really builds itself up. And if we pass from the salts to the acids, for instance specifically studying the acidity present in the earth domain, in the watery, fluid earth realm, we have something that corresponds as polar opposite to what arises within us in the internal process of digestion, that is, digestion after food has passed through the stomach.

If we examine all these processes in earth evolution in so far as they represent a relationship between acids and salts—in other words what we observe externally nowadays in chemistry, in terms of the process that develops from the alkalis through the acids to the salts—then this sequence of alkalis, acids and salts encompasses what occurs in the earth-developing process. And this process is largely a negative electrical process. To put it more precisely, if we express the external, spatial nature of this process, which crosses over into the physical, from the spiritual into the physical, we can represent it diagrammatically as follows. From the alkalis passing through the acids to the salts an effect occurs which is basically only hinted at here in terms of its direction (see Fig. 18, red, arrow) but, expressed diagrammatically, is really a process of sedimentation. And if we express this process in reverse, that is, salts, acids, alkalis, we would have to keep removing this line of sedimentation. They would act in a compression-like way giving rise to opposite rays, a streaming out (see right-hand drawing, arrows). [See also Plate 7]

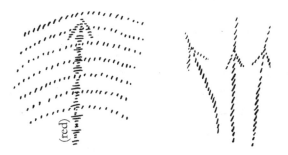

Fig. 18

And then we have here a positive electrical process. And I believe if you examine what I have drawn here, a diagram that is accurate, you will no longer be able to doubt the fact that this diagram is one drawn by nature itself. If you take a look at anodes and cathodes, you will find this picture inscribed by nature itself.

If we now come to the actual metal process, in other words approach the metals themselves, then we have in them something by means of which the earth 'undevelops'—as the opposite of develop, a word that no longer exists in our language but which nevertheless expresses a reality. It undevelops most in this way. And the metals do not tend to become increasingly preserved or consolidated in the earth realm but instead tend to fragment and splinter away. Thus they really embody the earth's undeveloping tendency, which is why they initiate a radiant action that is hidden from external observation. They have this radiant action everywhere. It is of very particular importance to observe this wherever we approach the realm of metals when interpreting nature in so far as it gives us medicines.

It is especially interesting to consider specific metals from this perspective. This view of things gives rise to perspectives that have been listed in simple form here in this table[25] as applicable to our mineral medicaments. To accomplish these things we had to compile everything that arises from a correct interpretation of this kind, and they will be accurate because we have initially only developed things that are based on a full and comprehensive interpretation of our observations. Here we can now also offer some interpretative help. For me it is really not a matter of just reeling off this table to you in some form. It needs to be amended and extended, and this must happen in the form of a written account. I am less concerned to recite this table than to guide your thinking in a direction that will allow you to see how it has, in fact, arisen.

If we consider the metals—or I would prefer to say 'metallity'—from this perspective, then we have what I described to you a moment ago as a radiant quality, present in diverse forms. We can find this in the form of something that radiates and streams out into the cosmos, destroying what is earthly. This is particularly true of the action of lead. We could say that through the action of lead, forces are implanted in our organism that seek to fragment and scatter us out into the world. This is implicit in the action of lead, this urge to fragment and scatter into the world, and so we can best regard this action as a radiating one. Radiant actions appear in a different way in other metals, for instance magnesium. This can be very clearly discerned. Magnesium's function in respect of our teeth is based on this. The action of a metal must pass through the human organism to unfold its effect. This is also what occurs. It is then a matter, however, of the radiant effect in turn undergoing a metamorphosis. And when the radiant quality initially undergoes a metamorphosis it becomes something I would describe as follows: the stream is now only direction, and what occurs is really a pendulum swing around the direction—an oscillation.

Such actions are ones we must observe in states of both sickness and health. In a healthy person these radiant actions are present as, if you like, the residues of pre-birth existence, of pre-existent life in the sense organs' radiant streams. They are always present. What rays out in the sense organs are the actions of lead, basically, in which lead is no longer present. And in all sensory activity throughout the organism, these streams or radiant actions occur. Nerve activity, nerve function, is largely based on attenuation of sensory activity in this direction, in other words involves a weaker stream.

From this you can see why I said, in my book *Riddles of the Soul*,[26] that neurosensory activity is hard to describe, since it would be necessary to preface such an account with all I have now presented here.

This oscillating, pendulum impetus, in which only the direction of a radiant current is still preserved, is something that underlies all respiration, all rhythmic activity in general, in the functions of the human organism. Rhythmic activity is based on developing this oscillation of movement, on a form of motion that is more inwardly consolidated than the radiating stream. For instance, in the group of metals or the realm of metallity, tin largely has such a movement. This is what makes high potencies of tin so beneficial: fairly high potencies for treating everything relating to the rhythmic system. Then, however, this radiant, pendulum movement can be further modified. This third modification is of very special importance. It maintains both the direction and the oscillation but only, in a sense, in latent form. But on the other hand it consists of a continual forming and dissolving of spheres which develop and undevelop in the direction of the current or stream.

What acts in our metabolism is based on these forces. And amongst the metals, iron is what unfolds these forces to a particular degree. This is why iron in the blood counteracts metabolic action as a third metamorphosis of the radiant action. In the case of the first metamorphosis, the action is directed particularly to all that relates organically to the I. With the second metamorphosis the action is organically directed to all that is connected with the astral body. And the third metamorphosis exerts its organic effect on all that relates to the ether body (see Fig. 19). [See also Plate 7]

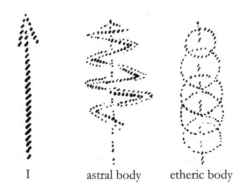

Fig. 19   I   astral body   etheric body

But now let us go further. What develops there as this ongoing stream of spheres, if I can put it like that, must—since in a sense it works down from the upper to the lower organism—continually be received. It only goes as far as the etheric—only as far as the etheric! But now the physical body must receive it through a force that works in polar opposition, for this forming of spheres must be met from without by something that enfolds and envelops them. Something must envelop these spheres (see Fig. 20). [See also Plate 7]

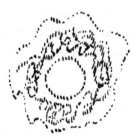

Fig. 20

This enveloping action can be such that it is more or less in equilibrium with the sphere-forming action. Under normal conditions this is of course due to the fact that everything working from above downwards is balanced by what works from below upwards. And this state of balance occurs particularly in the movement of the heart. But if this particular balance is uspet, then Aurum is the balancing metal to use. This re-establishes balance between the encompassing action and what is present there in the middle. Aurum can be used in circulatory and respiratory disorders for which there are no other concomitant symptoms that present follow-on effects. Where the causes of disorder are not found to lie elsewhere in the organism, we can use Aurum. If we notice, however, that the causes of disorder arise from a region other than, say, the boundary between the lower and upper organisms, then we must see that the more etheric, spiritual process unfolding there is not being met within the patient by sufficient enveloping substance processes. And if the activity we find there lies in digestion beyond the intestinal walls towards the interior organism—expressly beyond the intestinal walls— then copper must be used to promote this enveloping process. This takes us to the mode of use for copper, which you will also find amongst our medicines, and which is indicated in cases of malnutrition that present as malnutrition-related circulatory disorders. If we are faced with circulatory disorders that are not to be regarded as a consequence of malnutrition, then we give Aurum; if circulatory disorders are caused by malnutrition, then Cuprum is called for.

Now, counter-processes to the other radiant processes must also of course exist—material counter-processes to etheric-spiritual processes. When the process we must now regard as an inner process, causing this pendulum swing, the oscillation, becomes abnormal, when it becomes too strong, it can be chiefly observed in all that lies towards the exterior, on this side of digestion, in assimilation by the intestine of what has been ingested. Also everything that occurs in the realm of sexuality, for instance, radiates out of a person like this (see Fig. 19), somewhat resembling the staff of Mercury. The Mercury staff or caduceus derives from this—such things played into the development of these so-called symbols. What is at work here must be opposed, if it is not to burst its bounds, by the formative material forces that keep it in check and stop it from getting out of hand. These are largely to be found in mercury; and thus we can indicate a domain where it is really extremely important to connect what I said in the previous course with what we are now exploring in a more inward direction. If you connect these two aspects with each other, you will then have the whole process. This is something, now, that plays entirely into the astral, which arises there through the pendulum swing of radiant movements I described, and through the corresponding counteraction. This goes right into the astral (see Fig. 19).

But now, however, we may also need to engage with the actual radiant process itself, which is of course present in the human organism in the most manifold forms. On the one hand we find this in everything that acts by radiating out through the skin, and also has this direction of radiance in it. But we also have this process in everything of a diuretic nature, everything in us that acts to evacuate or expel. Just as, in gastrulation during the embryonic process what is outermost turns innermost, so here in this radiation we see something that equally works outwards through the skin and in a sense then reverses direction in the urine-forming process, in the process of evacuation. Whereas in polar phenomena we usually find something manifesting in an opposite direction, on this occasion we find something that is opposite in one sense and yet is of the same nature. We should never see the world in schematic ways. As soon as we proceed from theories, errors invariably creep in. It is impossible to adhere to a theory and not succumb to error. If, for instance, someone were to state that polarity is at work in the world, and to construct a schema, a formula for this law of polarity, dictating how polarity works, he would be able to explain one set of phenomena but would find his schema did not accord with another. If only people would see through the terrible tyranny of theoretical supposition in science! Of course we need to attempt to formulate theories, for without them we could never encompass phenomena at all. But we must also be willing to depart from our theories again wherever this is called for, and to penetrate into the domain where our theory no longer holds true. This must also be taken into account in conventional science. If we wish to propound evolutionary theory in an external, exoteric sense, we should follow external evolutionary theory and simply reshape it accordingly and so forth. If we wish to understand the human being from within, we have to take our guideline from what anthroposophy offers. Neither an anthroposophical nor an anthropological theory can be handled other than by departing from it when necessary and entering a different domain. But in what we call anthroposophy here, of course, we must enter the sphere of soul and spirit and from there return again to external, sensory phenomena. This path, you can observe, is one I pursued in an entirely independent way in my early books and in subsequent works, and now I try to include the other aspect as well. Fools will of course find these books to be riddled with contradictions, and on this basis they mount their idiotic attacks. There are German periodicals, of course, run by people devoid of any judgement, which engage in idiotic, combative campaigns as if this were a serious discussion of anthroposophy. I don't know if you're aware that the name of one of these people, who mounted a thumping, half-wit attack in Diederichs's magazine,[27] *Die Tat*, actually translates as 'Mr Thumper'.[28]

But now we must consider what can be described, and what I have described, as a form of radiation. And we must also counter this action. We do so by invoking everything that radiates in a contrary direction, for instance in silver. Here, though, we must be clear that silver has to be used as an ointment if it is to meet and engage with the direction of radiance that issues through the skin in some form, whereas it must be given parenterally in some form if the other activity is involved, corresponding in some way to the direction of evacuation. This is a kind of 'direction guideline' for the particular way in which such things must be handled; for as much depends on the way they are handled as on the quality of a medicine.

Now, I would like to let these observations, which touch on our medicines, flow on into a few additional comments I will make in relation to questions that have been raised. If I have not been able to give a fully rounded picture today, I beg you to understand that this was due to lack of time. But I believe that if you pay attention to the method I will use in briefly answering those questions, you will see that I have tried in recent days to organize the lectures in a way that has led up to these answers. I'll start therefore with a very characteristic question that someone asked, which relates to something real. The question was whether there is anything in the widespread popular view—which is founded on something real that people observe too little and therefore frequently overlook—that menstruating women emanate a kind of flower-wilting force: that, in other words, flowers in their vicinity fade and wilt, especially if they pick them up. Now, you need only consider the view of the human being we have elaborated here to discover the inner cause of this phenomenon. Just consider that what works in the flower and enters into the flowering process strives upwards from below. This flower-force in us, on the other hand, follows a direction that strives downwards from above; and so here, certainly, we have a polarity between what is cosmos and organically oriented. You only need to picture how this normal upward striving into the flower is opposed by what moves down from above in us (see Fig. 21). [See also Plate 7]

Fig. 21

An equilibrium is needed here, as exists in us under normal circumstances. Now imagine that the descending forces are intensified, as this comes to expression in menstruation. These intensified forces work in opposition to the plant's flowering forces. Thus you can grasp this real connection, this strange connection preserved in instinctive modes of perception and traditional lore, and can discern it by seeing things in this way.

Now here is another question I have been asked: 'What treatment can be offered in cases of asthma which is caused by spasms, and presenting as a syndrome involving blood congestion above and ischaemia or exsanguination below?'[29] What does this condition tell us? This form of asthma means that the neurosensory process has slipped down into the breathing process. Excessive activity in the breathing process causes the sensory process to slip down into it. We must counteract this in a polar way. We have to work against it from the opposite side. In other words, what nature has allowed to pass from outside in must be counteracted with forces that have the opposite direction. You will achieve this if you introduce the acid process through the skin; in other words if you use carbon dioxide baths or other acid baths. This will have an extremely beneficial effect for patients with this type of asthma. In this context various further things can be used which you will discover if you consider the other aspect I have mentioned.

Now I was also asked about the rationale for something which—and this also was part of the question—has caused such astonishment and joy in our clinics, that is, milk injections to treat blennorrhoea. The fact that this is connected in a large number of cases with lactation can be gathered from what I have presented in this course in relation to lactation. If you recall, we identified a sensory process in lactation, but one that has slipped further down. I detailed the abnormality that occurs here, and naturally the product retains directional forces. Basically, this is a process in which what has occurred within an organ is perpetuated. If you inject it you can naturally counteract a process associated with fairly similar aspects. This is therefore something where a chance empirical finding, based on trial and error, has had an extremely ingenious outcome. It is generally very important to consider process metamorphoses. If we cannot discern how processes metamorphose, we won't really be able to properly assess the simplest conditions.

Then the question arose as to the real cause of colds—of all kinds of complaints that we summarize under this diffuse term. Here too, albeit in a different way from that cited previously, sensory activity is pushed down into respiratory activity. Secretions or exudations that occur in consequence are only a reaction to this. Here something occurs in the organism, situated more towards its surface, which continually occurs in the interior of the organism through the reciprocal action of neurosensory activity, and metabolic activity. This continually occurs within us. Once again you should not be surprised that we can treat these complaints by very simple means through compresses and suchlike, whereby we push a kind of nerve and sense activity in from without, to a place where it is not normally located. All packs, compresses and so on involve inserting a nerve and sense activity into the organism, one that is semi-conscious but not otherwise present.

Now I was also asked about the relationship between muscle forces and bone forces. As to questions relating to homoeopathy, I hope that what I have presented will largely answer these. Various other questions have also been submitted, and I must respond to them a little.

The behaviour of muscle forces compared with bone forces can be characterized by saying that muscle forces contain actions in full flow that have come to rest and died away in bone forces. Bones—not now in a generic sense, but archetypally, are certainly transformed muscles. For this reason it is nonsense to seek a generic connection between bone and muscles, or even between cartilage and bone, and some have rightly pointed to the difficulty of looking for a kindred relationship. Bunge,[30] for instance, has highlighted the problems involved in regarding bone and cartilage as cognate, although he did not of course identify the nature of this difficulty. Just consider a time when all muscle development has not yet reached the organic and visible stage (see Fig. 22, red, and also Plate 7)—and this is largely also true, albeit only in very attenuated form, in the case of cartilage development—where muscles and cartilage are still undifferentiated (light shading), and when, in this undifferentiated state, during differentiation, polarity takes hold of these processes. Naturally it will then be very hard to

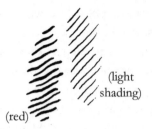

(light
shading)

Fig. 22 (red)

discern the metamorphosis. You can only discern an external, generic metamorphosis when its nature is such that polarity does not yet take effect in the transition of one into the other during differentiation, but the direction is retained. If polarity intervenes immediately in the differentiation process, however, quite a different configuration will of course occur, and will no longer in the least resemble the original form.

Some questions will be answered in the session immediately following this one. But I would beg you to regard the next question as one that takes us into an area where deep confusion can arise and where we should avoid drawing analogies. The question is this: Can one assign taste to a spectrum passing from sweet, bitter, sour, acidic through to salty, and perhaps also a spectrum of smells, and if so how? In relation to such things, specifically taste and smell, we really have far too few objective phenomena for analogies to be useful. Practical application of such things is of relatively little significance, for the moment we pass from the realm of the eye and the ear to that of taste and smell we enter a quite different realm. This is because, when perceiving visually, we are really involved with what is revealed entirely from the etheric domain, while the process of tasting and smelling is a realm strongly dominated by material processes, the actions of substances, metabolic effects. In passing to this realm of sensory activity, therefore, we can adhere to the more robust nature of what is expressed in metabolism.

Now I would like to briefly address a question that has a certain fundamental importance (other questions that relate to it can better be discussed in the following session). Without ingesting these substances, are we capable of synthesizing bromine, morphine, iodine, quinine, arsenic and other medicinal agents within us? This question actually takes us into profound depths of the whole human organization. We cannot in fact produce these substances, but we can produce the processes. While we certainly cannot produce lead within us, we are perfectly capable of producing the lead process within us out of the etheric realm, and then allowing it to radiate into the physical body. And so we can ask whether it might be possible to use this process homoeopathically to try to exert an effect on the ether body in such a way as to induce this self-metallization or self-radiating process, corresponding to a metal-radiating process. This can actually occur in a certain sense. But it requires us to gain close insight into the radiating processes that issue from metallity. You won't be able to approach these things, of course, if you remain stuck in allopathic thinking. But you can if, for instance, you consider the following. The process of dentition involves magnesium-radiating forces, or in other words forces that are of significance throughout the human organism, since the teeth, after all, are pushed out from the whole human being. If you now use a magnesium salt of some kind, let us say magnesium sulphate, and in doing so neglect anything of an allopathic nature, producing instead a particularly high dilution—here we will find it is necessary to use high, or indeed very high dilutions—then you will have two things. Firstly there will be the action of magnesium, which really ceases, however, where the teeth are seated. The magnesium forces do not usually breach this region in normal conditions. In a sense therefore we have to give these forces a strengthening impulse so that their action goes further and radiates through the whole human being. We can do this by using a salt, a sulphate in particular, for this conveys the magnesium radiation right through into the head forces. From here you can let them radiate back again. And this will in fact invoke a process that proceeds from the etheric realm—one that remains homoeopathic right into the etheric realm and involves only forces without any substance, having started with a quite different substance. You know that magnesium sulphate has already been empirically tested here, but we will only be able to use it in a rational way if we consider this whole context, for then we will see immediately, for instance, that the sulphate property is only half the picture. The other half of the picture is magnesium. And so someone who thinks that one could also use another sulphate will be mistaken. We will only mistakenly believe such a thing if we rely on methods rooted in the external world of the senses and on a rationality that only collects and combines sensory impressions.

To end, in relation to everything presented today, I would just briefly like to point out that we must, firstly, try to select isolated phenomena in order to delve behind the observed effects; but having done so we must in turn compile and interrelate all these things. In giving these lectures I have asked you—perhaps rather a tall order—to interrelate and gain an overview of everything presented. And now I would like to suggest one way in which things can be interrelated. For instance, someone asked me about Graves' disease. Here you could even look back to what I said in the first eurythmy lecture[31] when I pointed out that the thyroid is something like an incomplete brain. If you see the thyroid as an incomplete brain and become aware that the abnormal forces active in Graves' disease tend towards the thyroid and in doing so induce all the other symptoms which appear in the Graves' disease syndrome, then you will discover how you need to counteract this condition by means of something that, as it were, combats excessive head development in the human being. And then we are led in turn to the theme of our next session: we will find that we can exert a very beneficial effect on such things through purposeful movement, notably through purposeful movement accompanied by the speaking of consonants. You will achieve a good deal, in the case of incipient Graves' disease, if you make radical use of what we discussed in the eurythmy lectures. So there we have a connection, an interrelationship.

Now, rather than ending, we will conclude for the time being—apart from our next session—in the hope of continuing with these matters on another occasion.

After a short break we will reconvene and examine aspects that relate more to eurythmy.

LECTURE 9

Y OUR own knowledge of physiology and other fields must always inform the details of what I wish to say to you today in relation to eurythmy. This will come about quite naturally. But particularly when examining the kind of spiritual-corporeal process that occurs when we do eurythmy, it is unavoidable that I refer to deeper spiritual and physical relationships. And here I would like to draw your attention to the following.

We must initially consider the world process that occurs outside us, whose isolated details we usually only study rather than what is really active within it. Just consider that the earth develops in fact from a configuring tendency entering from the planetary sphere, and also from what lies still further beyond this sphere. The earth is configured from continually instreaming cosmic forces that manifest in distinct bodies of force as they radiate towards the earth.

In this context we can regard these cosmic forces—although they can in turn include everything I have previously said about radiating currents—as acting centripetally, and really forming from without what exists on and in the earth. It is actually true to say that the earth's whole metallity, all its metals, are not chiefly formed by forces of some kind in the earth's interior but rather that the cosmos implants them into the earth from without. These forces that work through the ether can be called configuring forces, generative forces working in from without. They stream in from the planetary sphere but not from the planets themselves, for then these forces would act centrally; and in fact the planets are there to modify these forces. It is particularly in this context that I would ask you to understand the generative forces. They are met by opposite forces, which in the human being and the earth absorb these generative forces and consolidate them, as it were gathering them around a central point so that the earth can develop. These can be called the forces of consolidation (see Fig. 23 below and plan on p. 120).

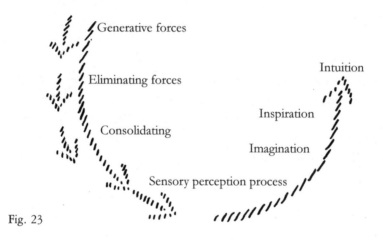

Generative forces

Eliminating forces

Intuition

Inspiration

Consolidating

Imagination

Sensory perception process

Fig. 23

Within us they are present as forces that shape and model the organs, whereas the other forces, the generative forces, are those which tend more to push the organs into the physical world from the spiritual, etheric world. This is a process we can gain a tangible sense of in the contrast between the pushing forces of magnesium and the rounding, shaping nature of fluorine forces. Once again, though, this process is one that comes to expression everywhere. It appears in the teeth from below upwards, rounding and shaping above, but also from front to back and from back to front, from above downwards and rounding off below. You can gain a further tangible sense of this process, for instance, if you picture pushing a spherical shape forwards, from outside in, so that a form arises, and oppose this with a sphere-forming process (see Fig. 24, red) that works from below upwards.

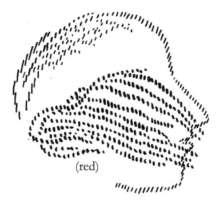

(red)

Fig. 24

Inside the form, between these two processes, you will now find a mediating element in processes of secetion, and then again the absorption of what is secreted by other processes and so forth. We can call all this 'secretion' in the broadest sense, for ultimately absorption depends on inward-directed secretion which is in turn reabsorbed. In between, again, there lies what one can best describe as processes of elimination.

You can again get a fully tangible sense of an elimination process of this kind if you imagine that on the one hand we have something that continually seeks to excrete carbon (see Fig. 25, orange) and on the other something that absorbs it again in carbon dioxide formation (light shading) through forward respiration.

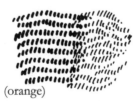

(orange)

Fig. 25

Then an elimination process of this kind continues there in a downward direction. And descending still further into the process of metabolism and limbs you have a consolidation process proper. But this con-solidation process is also present in the other direction. In the eye you can trace this again and get a fully tangible experience of it. The eye is formed from outside inwards—we find this already in embryology—

but is consolidated from within. What is formed is then internalized and the genesis of the eye depends on this. It is internalized (see Fig. 26, orange) so that in sensory perception we have this consolidation process as we advance towards soul and spirit in us, and thus to organs of spirit and soul, to the sense organs, in what is really an ensouling and spiritualizing process.

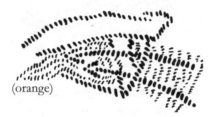

(orange)

Fig. 26

In a sense this is the descending process ultimately leading to organ formation (see Fig. 23 and plan below). Then, at the lowermost end we have the process of sensory perception, the perception of objects (see same schema). If this forms and develops further, towards consolidation, sensory perception becomes conscious in meeting consolidation, and becomes Imagination. When Imagination develops further and becomes conscious in approaching the elimination process, it becomes Inspiration. And when Inspiration develops further towards the generative process and comes up against this process to become conscious, thus penetrating it with vision, it becomes Intuition (see schema). One can develop this sequence of soul life from object perception to Imagination, Inspiration and Intuition.

> Generative forces
>> Intuition
> Elimination processes
>> Inspiration
> Consolidation
>> Imagination
> Sensory perceptions

But this process we develop in the soul realm also underlies the process of development and growth. As you can see here, it is merely the reverse of the developmental process. We encounter what has finished developing and ascend again in the reverse direction into growth. Generative shaping goes in a descending direction. We ascend in the reverse direction, going to meet growth so that what we develop as sensory perception and faculties of cognition in Imagination, Inspiration and Intuition is always counteracted by creative forces that come to expression in the generative forces, the processes of elimination and consolidation.

From this you will see that in the human organism we have the reverse direction of creative, originating activity, into which we enter when we raise ourselves to active cognition. You will gather from this that it is really true to say that what we achieve in Imagination involves the same forces that are active without our conscious participation in phenomena of growth, in formative development. When we rise to Inspiration we approach the forces that inspire us from without in breathing, that structure us as we breathe, informing the shaping forces and in a sense permeating and configuring them. And when we rise to Intuition, we are really ascending to the agent that enters into our plastic forms as substantial entity from the world outside us.

So here we see the human being as he is shaped out of the cosmos; and if we now apply the insights we have acquired through study of such things as anatomy or physiology, and cast light on them through what is given here, we can start to understand the organs and their functions. We can understand the organs and their functions if we see that what always works to shape and form us, what normally as it were entirely shapes and configures us, lives on the other hand as its other aspect—recall yesterday's lecture to understand this—in consonant movements which invoke unconscious powers of Imagination as I said yesterday, in a kind of streaming through the organism. So here you can understand how consonantal eurythmy engages with inadequate generative forces in us, deficient shaping forces, and guides them into the right kind of plasticity.

Let us consider a child in whom this shaping activity is inadequate, in whom this shaping plasticity is too strongly proliferative. This means that this shaping activity is centrifugal and, by virtue of this, makes the head large. In doing so, this activity prevents the head from imbuing itself with imaginative powers in the right way. These powers must be brought to bear, and so the child should do consonantal eurythmy.

A question was asked about a 'two-year-old, otherwise healthy boy with a large head, but not hydrocephaly'.

In consonantal eurythmy, when properly applied, you do indeed have a means to counteract this and remedy it. Here we come to the point where a thorough observation of morphology, the deeper aspects of morphology, shows that eurythmy treatment is indicated.

Another question was this: 'A boy aged twelve-and-three-quarters whose growth is noticeably retarded. No appreciable disease, but suffers with intestinal worms. Intelligent but easily tires of mental effort.' This is an extremely interesting syndrome, and all the symptoms point to a deficiency of imaginative forces and a proliferation of shaping organ forces due to insufficient inner shaping forces, shaping forces of the soul. These shaping forces of the soul, of soul plasticity, are also what destroy parasites. It is not surprising, therefore, that a lack of these forces manifests as worms. One should have him do consonantal eurythmy to address this condition.

These syndromes will directly indicate where you should intervene with eurythmy. Even if such signs and symptoms appear in a somewhat concealed form, eurythmy can still have an extremely valuable effect, especially when we also address the condition through medicinal therapy.

For instance, an interesting question has been submitted to me. Naturally I will have to respond to it in principle only. If complications develop, special note could be taken of them in a specific instance; but even if the condition in question is associated with other symptoms, from one perspective the characterization I will give here is accurate:

'I have a five-year-old patient who sustained a bullet wound during public unrest and lost a great deal of blood. Two years ago a deformity of the joints set in—conditions which later lead to anaemia and suchlike in adults. How should I address this situation therapeutically?'

Here you have a joint deformity in which the forces of plasticity are already working outwards, are no longer able to remain within and instead radiate outwards, departing from the patient rather than acting internally. Using consonantal eurythmy will make these forces radiate back in the most decided way. In consonantal eurythmy, you see, you invoke active, objectively active imaginations, which correct the deformities. In future, as the question already correctly suggested, people will show an increasing tendency to all kinds of deformity since they will no longer be able to form a normalizing human figure through forces that are involuntarily active. Human beings will become free, gradually also in relation to the configuring of their own form, but will then have to develop the capacity to make use of this freedom. In other words they will have learn to engender imaginations that invariably counteract deformity.

Now on the other hand, besides a lack of objective imagination, we may also find here a lack of objective inspiration which manifests—if I can put it like this—in a deformity of the rhythmic system. This deformity of the rhythmic system arises particularly where objective inspiration, which passes inwards, fails to engage with the circulatory rhythm in the right way. We can exert a normalizing effect here if we use vowel eurythmy. This vowelizing eurythmy, you see, acts upon inner irregularities which are not accompanied by morphological changes, in the same way that consonantal eurythmy works upon deformities or a tendency to develop them.

I have said previously that it can, however, be necessary to provide additional support if something like this appears in an especially radical form, as in the joint deformities we have just been discussing. Here we need to enlist therapy to aid the process of consonantalizing eurythmy, which works through Imagination in particular by stimulating the inner respiration of organs lying in an inwards-oriented position, from outside in, beyond the intestinal wall—that is, the lungs, kidneys, liver and so on. When we do consonantal eurythmy, then the occiput, lungs, liver and kidneys especially begin to sparkle and emit sparks. This really is something that shows the reaction, the soul and spiritual reaction to what is performed outwardly in the consonantal forms. In these organs we become an entirely luminous being, and the movements externally performed here are always met by movements of luminosity within us. With certain consonantal movements in particular, what I would call an entire, luminous reflection of the kidney's process of elimination arises. In this luminous process, in a sense, we obtain an image of the whole

elimination process of the kidney, which arises there through consonantal eurythmy. And then this works over into the unconscious
imaginations; and the whole process, where this part starts shining, is
the same as the one I described as subject to the influence of Cuprum. It
is the same process. And here we can point out to the physician that
there are, of course, people with certain forms of disorder such as those I
had a glimpse of yesterday—at least from a certain perspective—when
shown some drawings that had been much admired. I was shown these
painted designs and asked whether they testified to special esoteric
qualities. In a certain sense of course they do show esoteric qualities, but
it is very difficult indeed to talk to people about these things for they are
in fact objectively rendered kidney luminosity, objectively fixed renal
elimination. In this process of renal elimination, when it becomes
luminous in certain people of abnormal disposition, and when therefore
a certain stasis or stoppage occurs in renal elimination—thus a pure
metabolic disorder—the kidneys begin to shine. And when this special,
inturned clairvoyance develops, people start drawing like mad. Such
drawings are lovely, always lovely in an outward, formal sense. The
colours are always beautiful. Of course, though, people don't like it if
you say, Yes, that's lovely, but in fact it is your blocked renal elimination. I can assure you that blocked renal elimination and restrained
sexual longings—which in a certain way also culminate in metabolic
irregularities—are depicted by those with an especially mystical bent,
and presented as profoundly mystical drawings and paintings. We
should regard many of these kinds of things as symptoms of morbid
abnormalities that people are only just managing to live with.

Anthroposophically oriented spiritual science, you see, is not mysticism as many people understand it, for it does not entertain any illusions
about things such as those I have just described. On the contrary, it
undertakes research into these things. But people hold this against you.
They hold it against me that I have gone so far in public lectures as to
intimate—in this case in relation to poems rather than painting—that
the beautiful poems of Mechthild of Magdeburg or St Teresa are images
or inspired reflections of processes that arise through suppressed sexuality. Naturally people take it amiss when I characterize someone like
Mechthild of Magdeburg or St Teresa in this way. These were indivi-

duals with a pronounced sexuality which they held back, suppressed, precisely because it was too strong. In consequence certain processes of metabolism and circulation arise, which these individuals react to by capturing and fixing them in very beautiful poetry. Yes, viewed from a higher perspective, the phenomenon leads very deep indeed into the secrets of existence. But one has to raise oneself up to such a view. And therefore we have to have some intimation at least of these singular processes which shine out as inner processes when the outward movements of eurythmy are performed. And notably when what has been mysteriously infused into poetry is performed in eurythmy as I demonstrated yesterday, when a fine poem is first read out and then appropriately performed in eurythmy as we saw yesterday, either in consonantal or vowel mode, then this interlaces with the other aspect so that an inner, silent speech comes to meet what is outwardly performed in eurythmy movements. And if the process is not overdone in sensual poems but when, rather, it acts as accompaniment, a process of eurythmy accompaniment, to beautiful poems, then what occurs in a person is no longer a mapping of pseudo-mysticism but instead a real healing process. We can therefore say that by getting a patient to perform eurythmy movements in which he is urged to be awake, to listen and to attend fully to the speech sounds he hears, the whole phrasing of the lines, we enable him to rise to the external generative forces, the objectively intuiting forces. And it will be very good, especially with children and adolescents, to repeatedly urge the person doing eurythmy to attend very clearly to what he hears outside him. This acts on all that remains within us as residue of what materialism calls genetic inheritance—rather than what has unfolded between birth and death. A great part of this in fact is what we bring with us from pre-existence in soul and spirit, and by this means we can work on congenital defects, flaws and suchlike. By attending carefully in this way we can dissipate all the tendencies to fixate inwardly on what seeks to emerge in things like mystical drawing or poetry. Eurythmy of this kind responds after all to a beautiful, externally spoken poem and is the reverse process. A true mystic knows that an abnormality reflected in something beautiful is always partially suspect. By contrast, when we inwardly experience something that is beautiful in the external world then we cannot say that this presents itself to us in an especially magnificent, beautiful form. On the contrary, it becomes schematic, abstract, but abstract like a drawing, in the same way a drawing is abstract. But that is precisely its therapeutic aspect, that is what we want and seek. You see, if Mechthild of Magdeburg, for instance, had been able to do eurythmy to good poems, then she could have avoided her whole destiny as a mystic, and this whole historical saga would not have occurred. Arriving at this point, of course, we can say that good and bad cease in a certain way. This is the amoral sphere of Nietzsche, beyond good and evil; and of course we should not be so philistine as to suggest rooting out every Mechthild of Magdeburg. On the other hand, though, you can be quite sure that the supersensible worlds will take good care, as long as people do not let such things run riot, that appropriate relationships with the supersensible world are maintained.

Now I would like to try to clarify a few things, although we are running out of time. Firstly I would like to respond to this question:

'Would it not be possible to support therapeutic eurythmy exercises with rational breathing exercises? This would not have to turn into Hatha yoga.'

Well, I'd like to say the following here. Rational breathing exercises to support eurythmy exercises can only be handled in the following way in our era, given that human nature is proceeding ever further in a certain direction. You will find that vowel-based eurythmy in particular will tend to alter the breathing rhythm. You can discern this. And now we are faced by the uncomfortable fact of avoiding cut and dried rules, generalized dictates about what should or shouldn't be done. Instead we should first observe what needs to be done. In each individual case we need to observe this change in breathing of someone we wish to help, depending on his particular symptoms; and then we should draw his attention to continuing this tendency consciously. You see, we are no longer constituted like the ancient Orientals who could pursue the opposite path, breathing in a prescribed way to influence the whole human being in turn. This will invariably lead to inner jolts when prescribed or laid down in a particular way, and this ought really to be avoided. We have to learn to observe what eurythmy teaches us, in particular what vowel eurythmy teaches us about its influence on the breathing process. And then we can consciously continue what occurs, individually, as someone does eurythmy. Here you will certainly find that this process, this breathing process, can be continued in a certain, individualized way, in other words in a different way for each person.

Well, my dear friends, this is more or less as far as I can go now in answering questions. Due to lack of time, there is no real opportunity to discuss various things that have been left out. To conclude, I'd just briefly like to say, my dear friends, that you will have to be prepared for your medical colleagues to join battle with you the moment they realize more clearly that our approach is making some headway. You will need the conviction and persistence to dispel what you are bound to meet. The opposition you meet should naturally never cause you to neglect these things, but nor should we be under any illusions about the kinds of antagonistic forces we invoke.

Now the course is ending I would again like to say that, in order to make it possible for the movement to be inaugurated in the right way in the field of medicine, I will always abide by the principle of not taking a direct hand myself in therapeutic processes with patients. I will be on hand to discuss, consult and advise physicians, and you will always therefore be able to reject any unjustified intervention of mine in your medical work. I said the same thing at the end of the last course. This can become very difficult for me—I can't pretend otherwise—since anthroposophists look for this kind of intervention from me, and make all kinds of unreasonable demands. It is certainly true to say that anthroposophists, too, find it difficult to surmount their egotism. Sometimes, in fact, they can become even more egotistic than ordinary folk, and can even regard the greater good of the movement with complete and utter indifference. It is to the benefit of the movement when nothing is carried out in individual instances that the external world can regard as 'quackery' but that instead the whole of medicine undergoes a process of healing, undisturbed by any individual demands associated with personal aspiration. This can get very difficult, but we must maintain this direction, for in this field we will only make headway if we can publicly demonstrate something that is also true of the wider movement in so far as it is governed by proper understanding, and not distorted by those who fail to understand it. Simply by knowing what is happening in the anthroposophical movement, we have to be able to say that something held against us is definitely a lie, is quite certainly invented. In certain cases we must simply be able to repudiate such things. And we can do so if we are, as it were, inwardly initiated into all that is involved in stating, as I have here, that I myself do not intervene directly in healing processes but that treatment of patients, medical work, is instead carried out by the physicians who work within our anthroposophical movement.

Having said that, all I wish to add is that I hope that what I have presented here in this course—often only hints and intimations due to lack of time—will work on in you and come to due fruition for humanity's benefit. I hope that we will have an opportunity to continue in some form what we have now twice begun. Let us really try to do so. With this wish I will now conclude these observations, my dear friends; and I hope that our actions will correspond to our wishes in all these respects. I was very pleased to see you here, and it will be a very satisfying feeling to look back on these days that you have dedicated to enriching medical knowledge. The thoughts in which we are united will accompany you on the paths that lie before you, my dear friends, as you seek to put into action what we have tried to first elaborate here in thoughts.

COURSE PARTICIPANTS

Altemueller, Hans, cand. med. (dates unknown)
From Osnabrueck. Joined the Anthroposophical Society in 1920; in 1923 transferred to the *Freie Gesellschaft* (independent society)

Bachem, Max, Dr med. (?–1944)
Practising physician in Frankfurt a.M., specialist in physiotherapy and dietary therapy. From 1911 he was the deputy chairman of the Frankfurt branch of the Theosophical/Anthroposophical Society.

Brauchitsch, Georg von, D. Phil. (dates unknown)
Doctor of archaeology and a painter, from Danzig (Gdansk). He knew Rudolf Steiner personally from 1916/1917. Studied medical questions intensively for several years and took part in the course on the recommendation of Dr Friedrich Husemann.

Deutsch, Maria, Dr med., later Frau Dr Glas (1897–1983)
Physician in Vienna. Joined the Anthroposophical Society at the time of this course, and took part with great interest in the therapeutic eurythmy course that ran alongside it.

Deventer, Hendrik van, cand. med (dates unknown)
Studied medicine in Utrecht. Together with his fiancée, the eurythmist Erna Wolfram and her colleague Elisabeth Baumann-Dollfus, he instigated the therapeutic eurythmy course.

Deventer, Madeleine van, cand. med. (1899–1983)
Studied medicine in Utrecht from 1918 to 1925. Played a major part in initiating the Young Doctors' Course in 1924. Later collaborated with Dr Ita Wegman.

Doebl, Hans, Dr med. (dates unknown)
Practising physician in Munich. Knew Rudolf Steiner personally from around 1912.

Ederle, Robert, Dr med. (dates unknown)
Worked at the Clinical-Therapeutic Institute in Stuttgart in 1921. Wrote *Neue Richtlinien der Sinnesphysiologie* ('New guidelines in the physiology of the senses'), Stuttgart 1921, and 'Die Relativitätstheorie und das physikalische Weltbild Rudolf Steiners' ('The theory of relativity and Rudolf Steiner's view of the physical world') unpublished, 1920.

Fridkyn, Henriette Ginda, Dr med. (1879–1943)
Physician from Russia. Came to Dornach in 1914 and supervised the so-called 'Samaritan's Course' there after the outbreak of the First World War. Until 1918 she worked on the developing Goetheanum building, and also treated sick co-workers.

Glas, Norbert, cand. med. (1897–1986)
Studied in Vienna, and connected with anthroposophy from 1920. He was active in the anthroposophical youth movement. In 1939 he emigrated to England.

Grosheintz, Emil, Dr med. dent. (1867–1946)
Dentist in Basel. Member of the Theosophical Society from 1906. In 1913 he provided land in Dornach for the First Goetheanum to be built.

Grunelius, Helene von, cand. med. (1897–1936)
Was particularly connected with the anthroposophical youth movement and the young doctors' circle.

Hans, Hedwig, Dr med. (1896–1980)
Lived in Meissen.

Hermann, Max, Dr med. (born in Austria, died 1935)
Practising physician in Breslau, later in Munich. Involved in Rudolf Steiner's science of the spirit from 1907. In 1911 he took part in the Prague lecture course on 'Occult Physiology'. Collaborated with the medicines producer Marie Ritter in Breslau, focusing on the field of mistletoe therapy at Rudolf Steiner's suggestion. His studies on mistletoe host trees, on which he gave a lecture during the first medical course in 1920, were unfortunately not recorded in writing.

Husemann, Friedrich, Dr med. (1887–1959)
Specialist in psychiatry, member of the Theosophical/Anthroposophical Society from 1910. From 1921 to 1924 he worked at the Clinical-Therapeutic Institute in Stuttgart. In 1925 he founded a sanatorium that was first located at Guenterstal, Freiburg, and then moved to Wiesneck in 1930.

Jaerschky, Paul, Dr med. (1864–1941)
Physician for dietary medicine and natural remedies in Berlin.

Kacer-Krajca, Clementine, Dr med. and Dr med. dent. (1883–1939)
Practising physician in Mannheim. Encountered anthroposophy in 1919 through Marie Ritter.

Kalkhof, Josef, Dr med. (1886–1952)
Practising physician in Freiburg/Breisgau. Connected with anthroposophy from around 1919. Alongside his medical work he gave numerous introductory courses and was strongly committed to the Waldorf School movement, biodynamic agriculture and the threefold social movement.

Kehler, Walther, Dr rer. nat. (1875–?)
Chemist. From 1921 to 1924 was director of Kommender Tag company's Schwaebisch Gmuend chemical works (later Weleda).

Kiffner, Fritz, cand. med. (dates unknown)
From Breslau. Member of the Anthroposophical Society from 1920.

Knopf, Leo, Dr med. (dates unknown)
From Leipzig. Friend of Dr Roemer.

Knoeller, Karl, cand. med. (1896–1975)
Initially studied theology and then medicine in Munich and Goettingen from 1917 to 1922. Later worked as a physician in Hannover.

Kolisko, Eugen, Dr med. (1893–1939)
Member of the Anthroposophical Society from 1914. From 1920, teacher and school doctor at the Stuttgart Waldorf School.

Kolisko, Lilly (1889–1976)
Worked at the biological research institute in Stuttgart from 1921, carrying out trials suggested by Rudolf Steiner: 'Milzfunktion und Plättchenfrage' ('The question of spleen function and platelets'), Stuttgart 1922, and 'Physikalischer Nachweis der Wirksamkeit kleinster Entitäten' ('Physical demonstration of the action of minute entities'), Stuttgart 1923.

Kostytchev, Olga, Dr med. (1880–1956)
Practising physician in Moscow. In 1913 she gave up her medical practice in order to study anthroposophy in Germany and Switzerland.

Kries, Manfred von, cand. med. (1899–1984)
Studied in Freiburg, active in the anthroposophical youth movement. In 1924 was involved in instigating the Young Doctors' Course.

Margarete Mueller (1889–1980)
Nurse in Zoppot. In 1922 she married von Brederlov and became a branch leader in Danzig (Gdansk).

Noll, Ludwig, Dr med. (1872–1930)
Practising physician in Kassel. Personal acquaintance of Rudolf Steiner from 1902. Produced medicines with his brother-in-law Dr Otto Eisenberg. In 1911 he attended the Prague course on 'Occult Physiology'. From 1921 to 1924 he worked as a physician at the Clinical-Therapeutic Institute in Stuttgart. He gave medical care to Rudolf Steiner in 1924/25 during the latter's final illness.

Palmer, Otto, Dr med. (1867–1945)
Practising physician in Hamburg, connected with anthroposophy from 1908. In 1921, at Rudolf Steiner's request, agreed to take over direction of the Stuttgart Clinical-Therapeutic Institute.

Peipers, Felix, Dr med. (1873–1944)
Member of the Theosophical/Anthroposophical Society from 1904. A neurologist, he set up a private clinic in Munich in 1907, and worked there a great deal with colour therapy. From 1921 to 1924 he was a physician at the Clinical-Therapeutic Institute in Stuttgart.

Rascher, Hanns, Dr med. (1880–1952)
Originally a medically trained naturopath. In 1908 the medicines producer Marie Ritter introduced him to anthroposophy. In 1911 he took part in the Prague course on 'Occult Physiology'. Practised as a physician in Munich.

Rennefeld, Ilse, Dr med. (1895–1984)
Practising physician in Berlin. Frequently discussed treatment of her patients with Rudolf Steiner.

Ritter, Marie (?–1924)
Lived in Breslau. Producer of the Ritter medicines. Knew Rudolf Steiner personally from around 1907. In 1908 she asked him for advice about developing an anti-cancer medicine. Collaborated, in particular, with Dr Max Hermann in the field of mistletoe therapy.

Roemer, Oskar, Prof. Dr med. and Dr med. dent. (1866–1952)
Professor of dentistry, initially in Strasbourg then in Leipzig from 1918 to 1934, where he became Dean and then Vice-Chancellor of the university. Knew Rudolf Steiner from around 1908 and joined the Theosophical/Anthroposophical Society in 1910. Wrote a treatise on tooth caries which referenced the findings of Steiner's spiritual-scientific research (published Stuttgart 1921).

Scheidegger, Edwin, Dr med. (1867–1949)
Homoeopath. Founded the homoeopathic Merian-Iselin Hospital in Basel where he was chief consultant until 1937.

Scheidegger, Edwin junior, cand. med. (1894–1947)
Like his father became a homoeopathic physician and succeeded him as chief consultant at the Merian-Iselin Hospital in Basel in 1937.

Schenk, Leonhard, cand. med. (1899–1954)
Encountered anthroposophy during his student days and later worked as a physician in Nuremberg.

Schmiedel, Oskar, Dr rer. nat. (1887–1959)
Chemist. In his laboratory (established in Munich in 1912, and relocated to Dornach in 1914, as the germinal cell of what was later to become Weleda), he first produced plant dyes and later medicines.

Schramm, Hedwig, cand. med. (dates unknown)
Also took part in the first medical course.

Schwarz, Friedrich Karl Theo, cand. med. (1900–71)
From Mannheim. Later had a practice there as sports physician.

Stein, Walter Johannes, Dr phil. (1891–1957)
Member of the Anthroposophical Society from 1913. Gained his PhD in 1918 in Vienna with a dissertation on 'Historical and critical surveys of the development of modern philosophy'. Between 1919 and 1932 he taught history at the Stuttgart Waldorf School.

Tabuschat, Franz, cand. med. (1893–1927)
Studied in Dusseldorf and died young in 1927, from the delayed consequences of a war wound, shortly after starting to practise as a physician.

Tuyt, W.A.A., Dr med. (?–1944)
Worked as a physician and medical officer in Nijmwegen and Vlissingen. A personal pupil of Rudolf Steiner from around 1912.

Walter, Hilma, Dr med. (1893–1976)
Encountered anthroposophy during her student days. At the time of this course she was working as a volunteer assistant at a hospital in Mannheim. She later became a colleague of Dr Ita Wegman.

Wegman, Ita, Dr med. (1876–1943)
Member of the Theosophical/Anthroposophical Society from 1903. Ran a medical practice in Zurich initially, and in 1921 founded the Clinical-Therapeutic Institute. With Rudolf Steiner she co-authored the book *Extending Practical Medicine* (1925).

Zbinden, Hans Werner, cand. med. (1899–1977)
Practised as a physician in Zurich. From autumn 1935 was one of the four trustees

in the Medical Section's directorate at the Goetheanum. For many years he was president of the administrators of Rudolf Steiner's literary estate, and edited the medical books and lectures of Rudolf Steiner's collected works.

Zeylmans van Emmichoven, Willem, Dr med. (1893–1961)
As a young physician practised at Massord near Rotterdam. In 1920 he joined the Anthroposophical Society and was subsequently very active within it. In 1927/28 he founded the 'Rudolf Steiner Clinic' in Scheveningen.

No biographical information is extant in the archive for the following listed participants:

Mathieu, Dr
Bernauer, cand. med., Heidelberg
Weber, Gerhard, cand. med., Kiel
Schuett, cand. med., Hamburg
Hochuli, stud. med., Zurich

RUDOLF STEINER'S NOTES FOR THE LECTURES

For the second medical course
in Dornach, from 11 to 18 April 1921

(notebook archive no. NB 610)

11 April 1921

Head organization: It is an imprint of the

I, of the astr., of the eth. and an

action within the physical: such that <u>this</u>

phys. action is opposed to the forming of the earth and thus

dissolves

what is earthly; but at the same time what the earth forms

is within it.—

Hair   Silicon—: it dissolves plant substance—

Blood   when introduced it has a mineral developing

Urine   action—it differentiates the human being—

supplies form and development to the various

limbs—

it is in the blood, for otherwise the human being would be a

unity—

it is in the urine, for otherwise an excessive

egotism would occur (centralization of the whole system)

statt finden würde –

Im Haupte vermittelt es die Decentralisation –
dadurch ist es geeignet die Verdauung zur
Verwendung der Salze anzuregen. Es wirkt
auf das „Ich", das seine Wirkung dadurch
von den Gliedern aus auf den Stoffwechsel
ausübt. –

Kieselerde = Haare, Blut, Harn | hebt das
Kieselsäure = Haare, Knochen – | aetherische heraus.

Kalk übereingeschoben dann –
es steht das Astralische auf –
Die rhythm. Organisation = (Silicium stärker)
                              wirksamer

Das ist ein Abdruck des Ich in der Astralität
Kalk hebt das Astralische heraus –
es wird die Kalkwirkung stärker – sie ist
äusserlich (frei) –

führt man Kieselerde zu, dann vermehrt
man die Aethertätig – die dann
vom Organismus resorbirt wird und
belebend wirkt –

Wenn Müdigkeit – Schwäche der Verdauung –

führt man Kalk zu, so regt man die
Astralwirkung an und damit die
Absonderungen überhaupt. –

Wenn mit Kohlensäure – wirkend so, dass

In the head it mediates decentralization—

and thereby it is suited to stimulating

digestion so as to facilitate use of salts. It acts upon the

'I' which thereby exerts its action from the limbs upon

metabolism.—

if one administers diotomaceous earth then one

increases ether development—which is then

reabsorbed by the organism and

has an enlivening effect—

In the case of tiredness—sluggishness of digestion

Silica: Hair, blood, urine/lifts the etheric out

Silicic acid: Hair, bones—

Calcium in the opposite sense—

It cancels out the astral.—

The rhythm. organization: (Silicon more strongly

active)

if one administers calcium, then one stimulates

the astral action and thus

the respiratory rhythm.—

Here there is an imprint of the I and the astral

Calcium lifts the astral out—

the action of calcium becomes stronger—it is

external (free)

If with carbon dioxide—it acts such that

the blood rhythm is stimulated; and with phosphorus, such that

the respiratory rhythm is stimulated—

Im Havel =

Florin : Knospen, (annelz der Zöpfe, Haem der Mag.

Im dicksten Pflegt Ufen ründend =

Magnesium Knospen, Zöpfen, Haare, marginlaff;
Speichel, Mitag. —

In the head:

Fluorine: Bones, dental enamel, human urine

Rounding in the densest physical realm =

Magnesium: Bones, teeth, urine, gastric juices

saliva, milk.—

O_2 = ⅓ Sauerstoff : in allen Fetten und Kalkfigur —
sind bei Trennungs und Verbindungsprozessen Stoffe
bereitet nicht mehr brauchbare
Stoffe zum Ausscheiden zu.

H = im Wasser, in Eiweiß, Galle, Fett.
ausgeschieden durch (Amnios, Nieren, Galle, Leber.

Na. Aat : Lebensprozesse grundlegende Tierreich
ausgen. Fette und haut milchspärliche
in allen Teilen
Fettstoff, Harnstoff, Harnsäure

C : Zerstörung der Pflanzen Hilfsstoffe
Ausgeschieden in Galle, Calcium, Gallenleib, Fett
erscheint bei der Lebensprozesse

beim Ausgeschiedenem Ich — Tätigkeit der Atherleib —
Er ebnet den Weg.

Atherleib — wie er dem Astralleib erhält
→ Ich im Astralleib — schafft Astralleib
hват

Astralleib : entstehend : „Ich"

Ich —

O: 1/3 earth weight: in all that is solid and fluid —

serves to separate and compound substances

prepares no longer useable

substances for eliminating

when the I has departed—activity of the astral body —

It smoothes the way.

H: in water, protein, bile, fat

eliminated through sweat, urine, bile, air

N: azote: life-asphyxiator   Foundation of the animal realm

except for fats and free lactose

in all parts

fibre, urine, uric acid

Astral body—how it kills the ether body

→ I in the astral body—otherwise: astral body

fetches [?]

C: Destruction of plants   charcoal

endows colour in bile, mucus, gelatin, fat

engenders in living processes

endowing colour: decolouring. 'I'—

I

Chlor = C H Salzsäure
zerstört Miasmen

* Schwefel: Gehirn, Eiweiss, Faserstoff, Käsestoff, Haaren,
Nägeln, Oberhaut.
(verbrennt zu erstickender schwefliger Säure)
Schwefelwasserstoffgas giftig.—

Phosphor: phosphorsaurer Kalk:
Gehirn, Eiweiss, Faserstoff, als Phosphorstoff
Knochen an Kalk gebunden als Phosphorsäure

Fluor = Knochen, Zahnschmelz, Harn

Calcium: Kalkerde — Knochen

Chlorine: C H hydrochloric acid
             destroys miasmas

*Sulphur: Brain, protein, fibre, casein, hair
             nails, epidermis.
             (combusts to form asphyxiant sulphuric acid)
             hydrogen sulphide gas poisonous.—

Phosphorus: calcium phosphate:
             brain, protein, fibre, as phosphorus
             bones bound to calcium as phosphoric acid

Fluorine: Bones, dental enamel, urine

Calcium: Calcareous earth—bones

Potassium: (potash)—in the fluids/saps of plants and animals

Sodium:

Magnesium: Bones, teeth, urine, gastric juice, saliva, milk

Silicon: Silica: hair, blood, urine.

Iron: Pigment, hairs, cartilage, blood fibre.

chlorine compound in gastric juice

phosphoric oxide   chyle

organic compound haematin: blood corpuscles

Kalium: (Aschensalz) — bei Pflanzen und Tieren in den Säften.

Natrium:

Magnesium: Knorpel, Zähne, Haare, Magensaft, Speichel, Milch.

Silicium: Kieselerde: Haare, Blut, Harn.

Eisen: Farbstoff, Haare, Knorpel, Blutfasern.
Chlorverbindung im Magensaft
phosphor. Oxyd   Milchsaft
org. Verbindung Hämatin: Blutkörper.

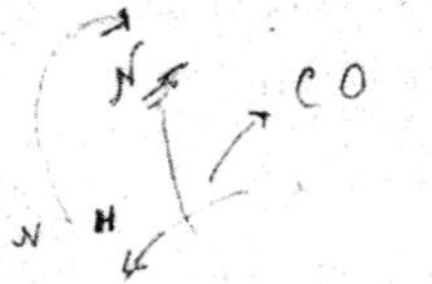

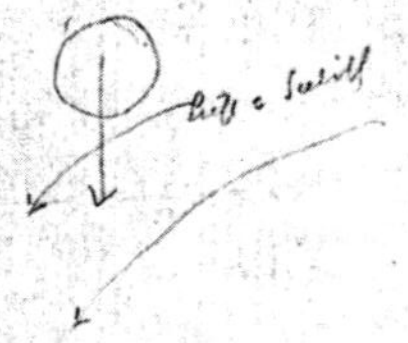

The development of the physical aspect depends on the composition

The spiritual aspect depends on the division, on manifestation of the elements

N   CO

N   H

Mech: within matter	embodied	In water: etheric
Phys: into matter		mech

chem.: into active force	ensouled	Through air: astral
Organ: out of active force		N: the soul
Soul: out of matter	through warmth: the I—	
Spirit: outside matter		cold: the spirit

Heat   eth.

Air   ← air: soul quality

Water

Earth

Nutrition: Into the structures created

Respiration—   by the etheric: the *

Neutralization of nutrition

Death: disease: I   astral.   Etherization in nutrition

Health. Birth: eth.—phys.   Astralization in respiration

Cure is a strengthening of the etheric   Before astralization, the astral reaches

Nutrition is etherization   the etheric: it incorporates an alien soul quality

When, before etherization, external ether passes to inner ether through the head organization—it impacts on the physical:

disease

---

* Translator's note: It is not clear what 'the' refers to or agrees with here. It is *not* 'neutralization'.

Sieht (schaut) man einen unterernährten Menschen, so fehlt die Befreiung des Aetherischen; der Stoff hält den Aether gefangen – der Mensch wird vom äusseren Aetherischen durchgiftet. –

Sieht (schaut) man einen arhythmischen Menschen, so löst sich ein inneres Astralisches nicht los von der Organisation – diese hält im Atmungsprozess das Astralische gefangen – der Mensch wird vom äusseren Astralischen – das in der Luft lebt, ~~[illegible]~~ verweicht.

Vom äusseren Aether wirken Wärme= und Lichtaether
Im Innern wird durch Aetherisierung frei gemacht
chem. Aether und Lebensaether –
diese werden im Gleichgewicht gehalten
oder: es tritt Störung des Gleichgewichts ein =
A. Wärme= und Lichtaether vergiften den chem. und Lebensaether.

Phosphor und Schwefel stossen den astral. Leib aus der phys. äth. Organisation heraus.
münden in die Verhärtung. –
Arsen – giesst den astr. Leib herein in die phys. Org.
mündet in die Erweichung. –

Antimon ausgleichend –

Im rhythm. Menschen kommt die Wärme unmittelbar an den Lebensaether heran – da muss Gleichgewicht sein zwischen den inneren Vorgängen und dem Leben des Kosmos. –

Phosphorus and sulphur eject the astral
body from the phys. eth. organization
end up in hardening—
Arsenic—draws the astral body into the phys. org.
ends up in softening—

Antimony balances —

In the rhythm. part of the human being the warmth ether comes
into direct proximity with the life ether—here there
must be balance between inner processes and the life of the
cosmos,—

If one sees (perceives) someone who is
malnourished, release of the etheric is lacking;
substance keeps the ether trapped—the person is
thoroughly poisoned by the external etheric.—

If one sees (perceives) a person with arrhythmia, an inner astral
is not released from the organization—the latter keeps
the astral trapped in the process of respiration—the
person is softened by the external astral—that lives in
the air.

Warmth and light ether act from the external ether
Within, etherization releases
chem. ether and life ether—

these are kept in equilibrium
or: the equilibrium is upset:

Warmth and light ether poison the chem. and
life ether

12. April 1921:

Das Ausscheidungsmoment des Astr. über ist das luftartige. —
Das Haupt ist für den Astr. dürstfällig — aber auf in
im Gleichmaßensystem wird Astr. abgesondert —

Im Doppelniftm System: für den Oberaxial dürstfällig —
luft zusammen mit dem aus dem Äther. für
werdenden Heilm. — fortwährenden Heilm.

C ⟷ O

Pflanzenwerden geht von dem nach dem — wird
aufsteigen — durch den Astr. Raum.
Nr. 3: da der Sitz des Kranklwerdens —
Die über der Erdoberfläche befindliche Welt:
für — Mensch als Astralleib — Es muss anders
allen oder Astr. angesehen werden als
von Innen kommend; alles was Erde ist von
oder von
außen kommend — dies einfachsten durch dem
arbeiten müssen

13 April 1921

The point of attack for the astr. body is the gaseous—

The head is permeable to the astr.—but also closed in on itself—

Astr. is separated off in the limb system—

In the rhythmic system: permeable to the astral—

Meets the astr. released from the living etheric—continual healing =

C ⟷ O

Plant growth goes from above downwards—is

stopped—by the astr. process.

There is the seat of developing disease—

The world above the surface of the soil:

Animal—human being as reflection—all

above/below astr. must therefore be seen as coming

from inside; all below/above astr. as coming from outside—this

maintained by the breathing process

Man atmet: dem Körper — abgeschwächt so, dass wir
dafür ist gefunden = alles, was die
Umgebung so erfasst, dann
man dem Tag über hat die
möglichst die Macht (Sommer)
auszuwägen — Es muss also so gefestet werden, dem
diese Schlafen im Sommer ist — Der Körper muss
lebend sein von dem, was ihn absolut annagt —
er muss und unten dem Leib/Köpfe prüfen:
(1.) den Köpfchen gleichzusetzen
(2.) die absonderlichste unwillste entsprechend so sein,
dann sie nicht empfinden werden —
(3.) Hunger — Durch dürfen nicht weichen.

Man muss Willigen herumreiten, die dem Menschen
zur Gift, sein auch. Wollen zur Geltung zu bringen,
doch ist gefunden, ist allem parallelösen fremd —
[das ganze ist der verschlafen Zustand] =
Willkürliche Symptome = Manz voller Einflüsse — nicht ord.
abhandeln —

1.) Vorab ungeordneten Körper
2.) die den gleich dem atmen
3.) die Erscheinungsamuläts

Krankheit erhalten =

Wenn wir den Mittelkörper der Sonne aus, so sagen wir in ihm
die Absätze der Wirkungen am Kraut als so verhalte am tut
machen gehen, um von unten weg den als des Pflanzezahn erhält -
Stickst man die Verhältnisse, unter denen die Pflanzenwelt
aufzieht, so hat man die, indem denen der Mensch atmen muss,
gewird so, dann seine Unterbrechungserscheinung vielleicht zu stark
werden — den schaffen sollten dass nicht aufzeige
zu denken — Vonspräch: so, dass über dem Irrthum
der außerordentliche noch glänzt — Hofmann vom
Sinneneinen

1) Inherited disposition: head

Causes of disease: 2) the environment through breathing

3) The composition of the earth

By exposing the middle area of the body to the sun, we stimulate in it
a reduction of the effects of the causes of disease. We make healthy
what acts upon plant nature from below upwards—
Studying the conditions under which the plant world thrives we find
those under which human beings must breathe,
but in such a way that his subconscious experiences are destroyed—
the rhythm. system must not begin to think—environment: such
that the extraterrestrial still 'has lustre' above the earthly—altitude
cures—sun cures—

We breathe: the cosmos diminished such that
Therefore everything is health-giving   an image of
that maintains the environment   the plant, not
in such a way that one has the   the plant itself
opportunity to make use of the night   arises
(summer) during the day—Thus it is necessary to sleep in
such a way that this sleep is an inner summer—The body
must be released from what astrally stimulates it—
it must remain under the influence of:

1) equilibrium in soul and spirit

2) breathing conditions must be such that we are not
   sentient of them

3) Hunger—thirst must have no effect

One has to induce effects that compel a person to bring his eth.
being to bear,
this is healing, is alien to all parasitic action—
[assimilating what has been allowed through =
The most important symptom: Difficulty falling asleep
          —not waking up properly

Man muß haben (in1haben): das absond. Lieb ist zu11 alle
an die Organe gewöhnen — ; man muß sie
lösen — man wird es dürch alles, was
über die Erde, nicht zu diese gehört =

Man muß alles aufzwingen: die absond. Lieb ist organein blick —
man muß ihn zu ihnen treiben —
man wird es dürch gehinden
geh1rigen Einkeün —

→ Bei den Erkrankungen des rhythm. Systems pfll
man gehörts dem zu1 anenwürden den
Ich u. Offr. einzuleib — der Auf. Phys. anderseits —
man hat nicht mehr wie beim Verstsystem die
Möglichkeit — durf (vorlesten — Wesson nepslein viel
zu hin, dann es spielt (vorlesten in Werfen hineinr
man muß die andern Erkrankungen von der
ein erkennen — man braucht eine zu1annunenr
fellung des Symptomes = die Sünden bei Verfollning

Die Heilung liegt in der Erzeugung von Reizpillen, die an den andern
organ1sein M1eller anforderungen stellen als die normalen. — Die
organis1n1e M1eller anforderungen müß erlebt werden —
K1rperl1ch Umanzimesten müß erlebt werden —

Die Erwartung der Seele — der Arzelin müß geh1ort1 werden —

Healing lies in stimulating processes which make greater demands on the lower organism than normal.—It is necessary to experience things that are physically unpleasant—

Awakening of the soul—the active must be nurtured

Difficulty falling asleep: the astr. body is too strongly bound to the organs—: one needs to release it—we can do this through everything above the earth's surface that does not belong to it =

Difficulty waking up: The astr. body is adversarial to organs— one has to drive it towards them — one will do this through a healthy spiritual influence —

Where diseases of the rhythmic system develop, we encounter interaction of the I and astr. on the one hand—the eth. phys. on the other—one no longer has the opportunity, as in the head system—to do a great deal through regulation of sleeping-waking, for sleeping plays into waking—one has to recognize the other diseases from that perspective—one needs to survey/summarize the symptoms: sins in relationship zur Umgebung – Atmen – die pumpen im Verhältnis zur eigenen Körperwärme – Circulation – Herzhorn – gehören hieher – aber auf der Innstange? und aufsondernd laufhäng – Milz – magen? Man wird kann sprechen noch nicht viel mit Heilmitteln, kann erst an mir dadurch etwas erreichen, dem man die vom Auseinanderschellen obwohl veränderten anwendet – also dem im Kochen, Verbrennen, Dämpflen – Duch magnetisieren

[Fernsicht Verhältnis: wie bezüglich der Kräfte da, draussen und grade Würzel näher lauscher wirklich aufzuwenden]

Was durch die Erdwindbeg gegangen – dann nach veränderl etwas Kochen, Verbrennen als rest die ätzung normaliziend an – was über des Erde bleibt – Wärme, kuh, Magnetismus etc reyt durchfalls die etwas eteng an –

to the environment—breathing—those in relationship
to the harmony of one's own body—circulations—heart disorders
belong here—but also the rhythm of nutrition
and elimination—spleen—stomach =
in <u>chronic</u> conditions not much will be achieved with medicaments,
and in <u>acute</u> conditions only by using ones
<u>greatly</u> altered from the extraterrestrial state
—thus through cooking, combusting,
transillumination—magnetizing =

[Fanatic raw food diets: only in relation to fruits etc.,
by contrast root decoctions are of important use]

What has passed through the actions of earth—then further
modified by cooking, combusting, etc, stimulates and normalizes
respiration—what remains above the surface
of the earth—heat, light, magnetism, likewise
stimulates respiration. =

Das Ich ist wirksam in der Blutbildung — zu
unorganischen von dem Blutrhythmus — im Übergang
vom Darm in Blutgefäßsystem.

Das Darmsystem ist durch die Vorbereitung — es ist
in den Organismus hineingebund — als metamorphosierte
Sinnessystem — geht auf Schmecken, wie Ahnen auf
Riechen und Hauptsystem auf Sehen —

Es steht im Zusammenhang des stoff-abg. Verhältnis —
zu tun mit dem Blutbildungssystem —

Das chem-phys. Verhältnis zu kosm. Horizontal —
und dem Rhythmischen System —

Das organisch- vegt. Verhältnis zum Kosmos mit dem
Kopfsystem (vert.)

Verhältnis = die Empfindung, dann die
○ Immerwelt anregt — es wird der
Rhythmus in die Dunkelheit versetzt —
der Ich zieht sich von der phys. Org.
zurück :

Empfindung = Die Außenwelt regt an; es wird
der Rhythmus erregt —

Need: sentience that is stimulated by the

interior world—rhythm is transposed into darkness—

the I withdraws from the phys. org. =

Sentience: The external world stimulates; rhythm is

stimulated—

The 'I' is active in haemopoiesis—must be distinguished

from the blood rhythm—in the transition from the intestine

into the vascular system.

The intestinal system is the preparation for this—it is built

into the organism—as metamorphosed sensory system—

relates to tasting as breathing does to smell and the head

system to sight—

The stat-dyn relationship to the earth is connected with

the haemopoietic system—

The chem.-phys. relationship to the cosm. horizontal

with the rhythmic system—

The organic-autonom. relationship to the cosmos with the

head system (vert.)[ical]

Müdigkeit - Mattigkeit - beim Treppensteigen

unlustig zur Arbeit zu Vergnügungen - einsamkeitssüchtig

geneigt zum Schlafen =

Hautbleichheit und Schleimhaut - wachsartiger Glanz u. grünlich.

zarte Teint der Blondinen - Lippen

Zahnfleisch - Mundschleimhaut - innere Fläche der Augenlider

Hände - Füsse - frösteln. (Mangel an roten Blutkörperchen)

Das Weisse im Auge bläulich

An Händen und Busen schimmern Venen in violetter Farbe.

Diagnose durch Geräusch in Jugularvenen - rechte und linke Seite des Halses --- entsteht auch bei starker Seitwärtsbewegung des Halses hinter dem Brustbein - Schlüsselbeingelenk.

→ Kurzatmigkeit, Gähnen, Seufzen - #: es ist zu wenig Einwirkung des von dem Ich aus durch die Stoffe - das Ich hat nicht genug Gewalt bekommen über die Stoffe

Man hat es vom 9½ Jahre an mit dem Wirken des Ich im Kopfe zu tun - es wird da dieses ganze unten = oben des „Ich" entfaltet -

Tiredness—weariness—while climbing stairs

lack of desire for work for amusements—hooked on solitude

inclination to sleep =

Pallid skin and mucus membrane—waxy sheen—delicate

greenish complexion in blonds—lips

Gums—oral mucosa—inside of eyelids

Hands—feet—shivering. (Lack of red blood corpuscles)

The whites of the eyes bluish

Blood vessels shimmer purplish on hands and bosom

Diagnosis through murmur in the jugular vessels left and right

sides of the neck—also arises through sudden sideways motion

of the neck posterior to the sternoclavicular articulation

Shortness of breath, yawning, sighing—#: there is too little I

action pervading substances—the I has not gained enough

power over substances.

From 9½ years onwards we find an activity of the I in the

head—this whole below-above aspect of the 'I' develops

here—

Cravings for chalk, coffee beans—   [acidity
                                          Gastric catarrh
                                          Mucal vomiting
                                          Constipation
                                          Cramps
                                          Hysteria, St Vitus' Dance.

depending on whether there is too little menstrual flow
  or too <u>much</u> — — — the head rejects
  the action of the I—or the
  pelvis does not carry it out—
<u>curable</u> if it does <u>not</u> pass into the chest,
  and has thus seized hold of the astral body.

Iron—fluoride chlorosis: 1-2 Dec. ???

Phys. rest   fresh air
Avoiding usual work, walks   nutritious food, not too much
sufficient sleep
pleasant, suitable activities

Ein Heilmittel ist als das jenige, oder von dem
Schlafenden Ich und astralleib nicht erreicht
wird, das sich diesem entgegenstellt — das
als Mineral wirkt —

A medicine defined as something that

is <u>not</u> achieved by the sleeping I and astral body,

that opposes these—that acts as a mineral—

15 April 1921

Arsenic—brings the astral body towards the phys. organs.

Warming—in the stomach area—

Habituation.—easy breathing. better nutrition.

Metabolism restricted— [in persons who need

release of the astral body from

the I]

Corpses well preserved

\# The I remains alone with the reciprocal relationship to the

external world—we have undermined mineralization.—

Magnesia usta

\# There is an irradiation process—which neutralizes the

mineralization process

Dysentery:

Diarrhoea, fever

Tenesmus

Evacuation: mucal—in lumps—streaks of blood

Pale pink jellies—serum-type fluid with

intestinal scrapings—bad: pure blood =

large quantities of protein =

(Drinking) water: in the organism an activity

of the astr.—I is undermined.

Diet. Arsenicum album 3–5 x

Diphtherie

Kinder von 2–4 Jahren – # die Prophylaxe stimmen [an] den Spendessinnes. Der
astralleib gibt von unten nach oben

Die Organe werden durchorganisiert
erhaltlich. Der Rachen wird
vom astral. Leib durchdrungen –

Pilzbildung –

Mercurius cyanatus 4.–6.– [hilft]
Mercur [fällt] dem Astr. zurück im wahren Menschen.

Die Auffassung: Die Personen werden bekommen genötigt
in sich auf die astral. Stoffwechsel zu
nehmen.

Im Astralleben werden die Organe
vom Astr. Leib durchdrungen dafür
mineralisch und vegetabilisch [frei] –
im Rachen
Man kann mal dann bis, wenn man
[Quecksilber]CN = indem man die Stoffe [kräftigt]
und Mercurius vermag – den ganzen
Menschen [in] einem [Zahnpilz] macht –
Im Stoffwechsel erhält [H] [Arbeit] dem
Astr.-H – [erhält] kommt man [zu] dem
Oxygen – eine natürliche [zu] Stoffwechsel-
[Beziehung] des Zahnes [beziehungsweise] – die
[an den Organen] von unten verschiebt [H]
[am Organ] – Cyan[id]

Diphtheria

Children from 2–4 years—#

phenomena accompanying learning to talk. The astral body passes from below upwards. The upper organs are permeated with astrality. The pharynx is pervaded by the astral body.

In arsenization the organs are penetrated by the astr. body, therefore they mineralize and vegetabilize—this can be remedied by falling back—via increasing power of radiation with magnesia,—making the whole human being into something toothlike—

Fungal growth—

In rock forming

In the maturation process the etheric body withdraws from astr. -I—thus remedied by arsenic—and notably in compresses.

In places where in water content of the earth

Diphtheria the process accompanying dentition—the astral activity from below strengthens—fungal growth [at locations where fungi form]

Mercurius cyanatus 4–6 x—| higher
Mercury holds the astr. back in the lower human organism

Infection: People become particularly inclined to react within themselves to the astral constitution

In phosphorization: the I activity bears the phosphorus—it must not fall away as otherwise the organism destroyed

Phosphor · nur als solches giftig –

nicht als Säure nicht

Zerfall der Eyweißheim.

plötzl. Entladung der ausgesprochen Muskelkräften –

Auflösung der Blutkörperchen.

Blutkörperchen · die erhitzten den "24" enthalten
Blut — Anämie

Nachweis der Untersuchs.

Verbessen in 24 – 36 Stunden. — aber trotzdem kann hinaufsteig —
Anfteigung —

gelblich gefärbt, [Cholesthesin], [Fettkügelchen] ausgeschieden
Belirien oder Schrimmfstoff

(Parakresse
Anämie

Phosphorus: only toxic in pure form —

                   not as acid

                   Degeneration of epithelia.

                   fatty degeneration of striated muscle fibres—

                   dissolution of blood corpuscles

Blood corpuscles: containing images of the 'I'—anaemia

        Necrosis of the lower jaw.

Improvement in 24–36 hours—but will nevertheless recur—

Jaundice, cerebral symptoms   (Headache, insomnia

                               delirium or narcolepsy

                               paralysis)

                               anaemia

Im Größeren wird fortwährend der Mensch eingegliedert ofer die beiden ebenen Systeme — im Begrenzteren wird dem das Abbild entgegengehen — oft gewerblich also mit das Abwegsystem — durch O —

Ortwechsel form. bittet die Wechselwirkung von X und? Symbol (etwa Bild Körper) in die äusseren organische Stationen, wo der aktuellere zu wollten Raum.

Menschkräfte hier dies um so mehr, je mehr Sie in sich Kräfte erhalten —

Towards imprint

Towards immediate
reality

The will sphere
vanishes in the

Here one must
achieve effects
with the sensory
sphere lying close
to the min[eral]—
on the blood

I. Astr.[al body]

Metabolism is
conducted upwards
Phys./etheric body

The will sphere remains
present in the sensory sphere
Here we must achieve effects
with what lies close to the
animal realm
on the nerve

In nutrition we are continually engaged without the two upper
systems—in replication the image is held up to this—but
usually only the respiratory system—with O

Potentilla Form.[osa] conducts the reciprocal action of I and I
image (red blood corpuscles) into the external organic
parts where the astral body can act from the I.

Plant saps do this all the more, the more they contain
earthly forces

Sensory activity is
conducted downwards

H²O

HCl : Magensaft 0·2% − 0·3%

+ NH³ : Blut (wenig), Harn, Ausatmungsluft?

H²S = Darmgase

NaCl = Blut, Geschäfte, Harn.

KCl = Blut, Muskeln, Milch, Harn

salmiak NH₄Cl = Harn

+ CaCl₂ = Harn, vielleicht Knochen

CaFl₂ = Knochen, Zähne

CaSO₄ = } Geschäfte
Na₂SO₄ = }

NaH₂PO₄ (Harn)

Na₂HPO₄ } Geschäfte
Na₃PO₄ }

KH₂PO₄
K₂HPO₄ } Geschäfte
K₃PO₄

Ca(H₂PO₄)₂
CaHPO₄ } Knochen
Ca₃(PO₄)₂

Mg₃(PO₄)₂ Knochen
+ NH₄MgPO₄ Harn
    SiCO₄ Haare

P darf übh in den Geschäfte
S darf sowohl in   „

Das Calcium in den Knochen
  „ Magnesium „   „

Die anorganischen Verbindungen : Ich. —

An dem N die Entwicklung des Lebens gebunden

H$_2$O:

HCl: Gastric juice 0.2%–0.3%

NH$_3$:   Blood (little), urine, expired air

H$_2$S: Intestinal gases

NaCl: Blood, tissue fluids, urine

KCl: Blood, muscles, milk, urine

Ammonium chloride NH$_4$Cl: Urine

CaCl$_2$:	Urine, perhaps bones			
CaFl$_2$:	Bones, teeth	KH$_2$PO$_4$		
CaSO$_4$:	Tissue fluids	K$_2$HPO$_4$	tissue fluids	
Na$_2$SO$_4$:		K$_3$PO$_4$		
NaH$_2$PO$_4$:	(urine)	Ca(H$_2$PO$_4$)$_2$	bones	
Na$_2$HPO$_4$:	Tissue fluids	CaHPO$_4$		
Na$_3$PO$_4$:		Ca$_3$(PO$_4$)$_2$		
		Mg(PO$_4$)$_2$	bones	
		NH$_4$MgPO$_4$	urine	
		[????] hair		

P   through 'I' in tissue fluids

S   through the astral body in " "

Calcium   in bones

Magnesium   "   "

Inorganic compounds: I—

Asphyxiation of life tied to N

Elemente:
O — Aufbau der Kohlenwasser... ...
H — ...
N — ...
C — als ... bei Pflanzenaufbau ...

Cl
S
P / H
Ca
K
Na
Mg
Si
Fe

Elements: O   Cause of combustion and fermentation processes—

H   Decomposition product of foods

N   Life asphyxiator

C   as charcoal when plants are destroyed

Cl

S

P

Fl

Ca

K

Na

Mg

Si

Fe

Protein Körper Eiweissstoffe — noch gelöst als nothwendig:
— Material des Gebäude Zuwachs.

Fette: Heizmaterial — Verbrennung =

Kohlehydrate — zum Aufbau ? gehen zu in das Leben
Heizmaterial —

Salze

Wasser ½ des Körpers

Chlorophyll Einverleibung # der Lebenskräfte

Chlorophyll
Einverleibung — wachsender Eiweis — N

Assimilation = machen = Motive
mittel Rhythmus
⅜f , Nerven-Bewegung = die äusseren
Kräfte —

Einverleibung = Fett —

Stoffwechsel

Proteins = quickly decomposed as nutrient = living protein stable

Fats: fuel—combustion =
Carbohydrates—only glycogen in the liver for constructive synthesis
                                                    fuel

Salts
Water $^2/_3$ of the body

Chlorophyll   Protein synthesis # the life ether dissolves protein, which is coagulated out through the chem. ether and permeated with light and warmth. The fats and carbohydrates with warmth the protein—with light—

the movement of the ether to the cells from tissue fluid—

to what purpose? Tissue fluid—alternating protein—N

free of N

Doses: low: metab.
 " " medium: rhythm.
 " " high: neurosensory realm = external
                                        forces

Injections: curtailed forces are
                   introduced—rejuvenating
Embrocations: fat—

The internal organs breathe: tissue fluid
is bearer of the metabolism—
            N   the substances which through food
            O   water vapour are introduced
            C   then
      air   stored

The lungs at risk of becoming head: excessive predominance of
the I.
One must counteract this through external salt applications—Hg
internally

Softening of the brain—paralysis—

Psychiatric cases =

Metabolism ?

Not for Imagination—Inspiration—

a corporeal aspect there too

Inner developmental capacity

wanes—: injections,

embrocations—

different environment—

Diseases affecting brain and liver:

The reciprocal action such that the liver is at risk

of becoming brain, uses up too

much of it—Hg internally: external salt applications (calcium

salts)—

The nitrogen that is exhaled?

    # Maintenance of sensory activity

    and the inner spiritual activity

    of the organs—

? Phosphorus Sulphur: compress if they become elemental

? Carbohydrates, fats, protein—

? Left-handedness—etheric body man, woman

    # Astral body more strongly developed in left-handers

Der Stickstoff, der ausgeatmet wird?

    # Unterhaltung der Sinnestätigkeit

    und der inneren geistigen Tätigkeit

    der Organe —

2? Phosphor Schwefel = die Umschlag, wenn sie elementell werden.

1. Kohlehydrate, Fette, Eiweiss —

2. Linkshändigkeit — Ätherleib Mann, Frau

    # astralisch stärker bei den Linkshändern ausgebildet.

2. Farbwelhe bei Vokalen =

Die innere Einheit des Sinnen [...]

— Volbraus[...]

— Blumenverweichborn bei der Periode:

Erfaßung des inneren
Tätigkeit des inneren
Menschen.

Autun, der durch Volbrausfängen entspl[...]
[...]haft obern, Welt here

undere —

Kulturfauns Werke

? Seeing colours in the vowels. =

    # The inner unity of what is perceived by the
      senses

  Traditional views

? Withering of flowers at menstruation:

    # Inner activity of the lower human organism
      increased

? Asthma, due to spasms:

  Excess blood above, blood void below—

  Carbon dioxide baths

N Schneidezer:

<u>Weber Rosenberg:</u>

Bekämpfes der mannigfachen
Tastphänomenen?

* 1857 — 1888 Dresden — 96 und niederegd Berlin =
†)1907

Für Soethes Farbenlehre — Phästierung. — Zuteilung-
und Ingenieurwissenschaft?

leitende Spender = Energetisches psychisches Substrat. —

Grundform = Coffeinin =

$x = d \cdot l \cdot \ddot{r}$
Sinnsstein —

Vorm Energieformen — im Verzicht zu
erhalten Formen.

Dr Scheidegger

Iodine—Hg—P—As

Concerning Dr Rosenbach:

   Combated those who do not

   gather sufficient facts.—

* 1851–1888 Breslau—96 resigned from post in Berlin
  + 1907

For Goethe's Theory of Colours—move. of blood—infectious
   and ingestive diseases =

Governing idea: a pathology of energetic forces.—

Giamb.[attista della] Porta = Cohnheim. =

   x = d.i.

   Stimulus

   Disposition

Cosm. energy forms—become coarser forms in body

kosm. Energien während des Schlafes. =
_____

Religion Hamilton —

Bioenergol ? =
_____

Von den toten der Ashonga .

Cosm. energies during <u>sleep</u>. =

Religion [???]

<u>Bio-energetics</u> =

At the Gates of Spiritual Science

treibend

Wurzel

Wurzel von Enzian (Gentiana lutea) = { vom Kopfe
(Abkochung) – angeregen.

bitteren Geschmack } macht Reaction der versch. Organe
macht genug? } antewal. Anregung

gerbstoffhaltig = reg. Anregung
sehr Öel
=

Würzel der Nelke (ganz unbekannt) } vom Kopfe
(Abkochung) angeregen

Geschmack herb – macht reg. Anregung – die
aeth. Öel Nahrungsstoffwechsel werden frei
Stickstoff in Angriff genommen
Gerbstoffe

angeregen auf die unteren Abwerg.
stillt den Magen "
wirkt diese minundzhun
Hälfte Dampfnaphten fort
eigentl. Dafer Kopfschmerz

appetitanregend
Dyspepsie
unbeteiligungen?
Gift, Rheumatismus
siehen beim Darf.

Durchfall
schleimsteften der Darme

angeregen auf unteren
Magen = Spannungspunkt.
dadurch Darmtätigkeit
angeregen

Schwächig

Root

Root of gentian (*Gentiana lutea*): (decoction)	Drawn towards the head	Stimulates lower respiration strengthens stomach, mineralizing action gets rid of intest. parasites large doses headache	Lack of appetite Dyspepsia — stimulant Pelvic congestion Gout, rheumatism, anti-fever action
Bitter taste — strong reaction of ant. organs astral stimulus Strong smell			
Contains sugar I stimulus Fatty oil			
Root of herb bennett (*Geum urbanum*) (Decoction)	Drawn towards the head	stimulating effect on lower neurosensory network: thus stimulates intestinal activity	Diarrhoea — anti-fever intestinal mucilage
Taste bitter — strong I stimulus nutrients are engaged at an <u>early</u> stage ess. oil starch tannin			

Schwertlilie (Iris germanica):
(Wurzel und Knollen?) =
widerstandsfähig
billiges Geschmack
Herz
Harn...
Gesichtsinn

Kraut (Herba) =
Majoran (Majorana Origanum)

Auszug:
...

Wärmekräfte

Bearded lily (*Iris germanica*):	Induces strong I activity	diuretic purgative	dropsy
root decoction			
repulsive odour			
bitter taste			
resin			
starch			
tannin			

Herb (herba):			
Marjoram (*Majorana origanum*)			
Infusion:	Stimulates: astral body	diaphoretic acts on the respiration of the internal anterior organs	catarrhs colds uterine weakness
warming taste			
sharp bitter "			
aromatic fragrance			
eth. oil			
salts			

Wurzeln (Blüten):

Holländer Fieder (Sambucus nigra)
Aufguss
äth. Oel
Schwefel

Samen (Semen) Kümmel (Carum carvi)
äth. Oel
Auszug

Katarrh

Flowers (Flores):

Elder (*Sambucus nigra*)

infusion	Stimulates the ether b. (in reciprocal action with the astral body.	Acts on respiration of the upper posterior [lower] organs	catarrhs, held back perspiration, hoarseness, coughing (rheumatism!) spring
ess. oil		diaphoretic	
sulphur		purging	
		blood-cleansing	

Seeds (semen) caraway (*Carum carvi*)

decoction	strongly stimulates the I from the head	in enemas	stomach cramps
ess. oil		anti-irritant	colic
spice · wax		strengthens digestion	flatulence
smell · galactose		enhances activity of tissue fluid in head	deficient lactation
resin			

Pb engages the head's vehement generative activity:
thereby tissue fluid in worrying activity—uses up
a great deal

Lead: radiates: I—generative activity: imag.—outside

Tin: oscillates: astr.—inspiration activity—breathing

Iron: rounds: eth.—intuition activity—circulat. intuit.

Cuprum: eth.: inner eliminating activity —permeating
the body

Hg: astr.: eliminating activity inwards will

Ag: I. It invokes vehement expelling from below
activity upwards

A salt: such that it preserves
the action of earth

acids alkalis salts

acids neg. electr: they absorb

alkalis pos. electr: they eliminate
generatively

The metal—furthest from the
earth—it belongs
to the planet. sphere

Lead: stomach pain, nausea, vomiting of milky-white mass
Slowing of pulse—pale face—
Lips bluish, voice failure—
Sobbing; deafness—
Paralysis of lower extremities
Constipation (more rarely diarrhoea)
States of unconsciousness, narcosis
Convulsions
Antidote: sodium sulphate—magnesium sulphate

Lead colic— contracting pain in navel area
tension in lower abdomen
slowed pulse
stools retained
urine production stopped—
Lead cachexia: absorption of lead vapours gums slate-grey
wasting margins
slackening muscles teeth greyish-
livid face brown
coloration
emaciation

Fragen

- quantitative Atom in bringen zur Verdeutlichung der (ein.
  Erscheinung - Übergänge.

2 Erkältung (Katarrh): Entzündung = die Samentätigkeit
  wird in die Tätigkeit
  gestellen. (Absonderung) -

2 milch- Injection bei Blenorrhoea. - Meilung: es ist dem
  Absonderungsvorgang gegen
  die Absonderung.

2 harnsäurehaltl. Mittel. man hat die ... um ...
  werden zu bewerten.

2. Milz reichliche - Vermehrungsverfle.

2 Spectrum bei Geschmack - Geruch.

Bildung?:
Absonderung?:
Verhaltungs-:

Questions

? rational breathing exercises to support
    eurythmy exercises   eu.

? colds (catarrhs):   origin: sensory activity
    pushed into breathing
    activity (secretion)—

? Milk injections for blenorrhoea.—cure: using
    a secretion
    product
    to combat secretion

? homoeopath. medicines. one must consider the pol. action
    from above and below

? Muscular forces—bone forces.
? Range of tastes—smell

Developing:	undeveloping:	Ag
Secreting:	withdrawing:	Hg
Consolidating:	encompassing:	Cu

? Child lost much blood due to bullet wound

eu

Limb deformity. =

Cu

NOTES

Text sources: The present volume is based on shorthand transcripts by the trained shorthand secretary Helen Finckh (1883–1960), which she herself also transposed into full text.

The notes to the 4th German edition of 1984 refer to two different transcripts, one of which was said to be no longer extant but which had served as master copy for the first typescript. The first edition in the Collected Works (GA) of 1963 was then based on Frau Finckh's shorthand transcripts after comparison with the 1921 typescript. Textual corrections made at that time were marked 'according to the shorthand version' in the notes. After more careful examination, however, it became apparent that all previous editions were based on Frau Finckh's shorthand transcript. Lack of rigour when editing the 1921 typescript may have led to variations in the text that gave an impression of two different transcripts with slight differences between them. However, this is not the case.

On the other hand, a second shorthand version by Lilly Kolisko did indeed exist. Original shorthand transcripts, including the one for this present volume, were fortunately acquired by the archive from Frau Kolisko in 1977. Since the two versions use different shorthand systems—Frau Finckh used the Stolze-Schrey system while Frau Kolisko that of Gabelsberger—they can usefully augment each other where any difficulties arise in interpreting each transcript.

For the 2001 edition, the text was first carefully compared again with Frau Finckh's full typescript. Where there was any lack of clarity, the original shorthand was checked once more; and finally a few critical passages that could not be satisfactorily clarified were compared with Frau Kolisko's shorthand version. A few important passages were also clarified by comparing them with Rudolf Steiner's own notebook entries for the course. In some places the editors added words not contained in the transcripts, indicating these additions with square brackets. In each case the additions serve to complete an unfinished phrase or as clarification.

Eva Gabriele Streit MD and Doerte Mehrling carried out the editorial work.

The notebook: The notebook to the present volume (NB 610) was in the possession of Ita Wegman and, together with the rest of her literary estate, was passed to the manuscript collection of Basel University library. The administrators of Rudolf Steiner's literary estate were allowed to photocopy notebooks and memos by Rudolf Steiner in this collection and use them in preparing editions of the relevant lecture courses. Notebook 610 is particularly profuse and detailed, and has been reproduced here in full in so far as it relates to the present course.

Drawings in the text: These were executed by Assia Turgenev and Hedwig Frey based on sketches in the shorthand transcripts. Three drawings (on pp. 66 and 70) had to be redrawn for the 2001 edition by Doerte Mehrling because they deviated considerably from those in the transcript. For one of these a new allocation in the text was necessary. These changes all relate to the lecture given on 15 April 1921, for which, unfortunately, the original board drawing is no longer extant.

The board drawings (plates): All except two (15 April 1921 and lecture 2 of 18 April 1921) of the original board drawings for this course have survived since they were made on paper stretched on the board. They are reproduced in volume XXII of the series *Rudolf Steiner—Wandtafeln zum Vortragswerk* ('Board drawings by Rudolf Steiner'). At relevant points in the text of this volume, indications of the original board drawings ('plates') are given. Plates 4 (14 April 1921) and 5 (16 April 1921) were also used for the lectures on the same day that formed part of *Eurythmy Therapy* (CW 315), and therefore contain additional drawings that have no direct connection with this medical course.

1. See *Spiritual Science and Medicine*, CW 312.
2. Oskar Roemer, 1866–1952, professor of dentistry and director of Leipzig University's Institute of Dentistry. From 1925 he was Dean of the medical faculty at Leipzig University. Publication: 'On dental caries, with reference to Rudolf Steiner's spiritual research', Stuttgart 1921. He held many lectures on this theme, including some attended by Rudolf Steiner.
3. Albert Einstein, 1879–1955: The Special and General Theory of Relativity.
4. See *Goethes Naturwissenschaftliche Schriften* ('Goethe's Scientific writings') edited by Rudolf Steiner, in Kürschner's *Deutsche National-Literatur* (GA 1a-e) vol. III, The Theory of Colours: introduction, p. 88: 'The eye owes its existence to light. Light calls forth from indifferent animal organs of orientation an organ to be its equal, and thus the eye forms through light, for light, so that inner light may meet the outer light.'
5. Rudolf Virchov, 1821–1902, professor of pathological anatomy in Würzburg and Berlin.
6. Ernst Haeckel, 1834–1919.
7. Eugen Dubois, 1858–1940, Dutch military physician. Publication: 'Pithecanthropus erectus, a humanoid transition', Batavia 1894.
8. Edwin Scheidegger, 1867–1949, founder and consultant at the Merian-Iselin Hospital in Basel, which opened in 1918. A homoeopath by training, he remained loyal to this therapeutic approach throughout his life. He was a member of the Paracelsus Society. The lecture he gave during the first medical course (GA 312) is unknown and no transcript exists.
9. Moritz Benedikt, 1835–1920. His essay 'The Tuberculosis question' gives a brief survey of the social issues that accompany tuberculosis, and was published as a supplement to his autobiography, 'Aus meinem Leben', Vienna 1906.
10. Substances: this relates to the lecture by Dr Scheidegger during the first medical course, *Spiritual Science and Medicine*, CW 312.
11. Cf. 'Ruten- und Pendellehre' ('Dowsing rods and pendulums'), Vienna and Leipzig 1917, chapters IV and V; *Theosophy* (1904), CW 9.
12. See the lecture of 7 April 1921 in CW 76, *Die befruchtende Wirkung der Anthroposophie auf die Fachwissenschaften* (not translated).
13. Waldorf School: founded in 1919 by businessman Emil Molt for the children

of the employees of the Waldorf-Astoria cigarette factory in Stuttgart, and initiated and directed by Rudolf Steiner.

14. In earlier editions, the editors included the word 'not' and the phrase thus read: 'not yet entirely mineral in character'. After very careful examination of the transcripts by two experienced stenographers, a 'not' was not found in either of the two stenographs made by Frau Finckh and Frau Kolisko. It should also be noted that this particular passage was written very fluently and without problematic passages.

15. Ferrum muriaticum: muriaticum derives from the Latin *muria* and means brine. Salts formed from hydrochloric acid are substances containing sodium chloride, and are called 'muriatic'. The reference here is to $FeCl_3$, called Ferrum sesquichloratum.

16. See note 2.

17. See note 1.

18. Rudolf Steiner was aware of serum treatment. Cf. *Spiritual Science and Medicine*, CW 312, note to p. 114, p. 391 (in German edition).

19. See Goethe's *Faust*, Part 1, verse 1740 (Study).

20. This passage has gaps in both transcripts, and cannot be reconstructed with any certainty. The symptoms referred to can however be read clearly, as can the phrase 'anaemic conditions', and this is also proven by reference to Steiner's notes for the lecture.

21. As far as we know, no transcript of this lecture survives. However, one can see from Rudolf Steiner's notebooks that it included detailed discussion relating to Dr Rosenbach. See next note.

22. Ottomar Rosenbach, 1851–1907, physician and professor in Breslau and Berlin. He published a large number of books on physiology and pathology (e.g. *Grundriss der Pathologie und Therapie der Herzkrankheiten*, Berlin 1899). Rudolf Steiner's library contains a short treatise by Rosenbach entitled *Energetik und Medizin* ('Energetics and medicine') published in 1897.

23. Herb bennet: *Rhizoma caryophyllata*, rootstock (rhizome) of *Geum urbanum*. The German name for the plant (Nelkenwurzel) relates to the root's weakly aromatic, clovelike smell. The root tastes bitter and tart, and has an astringent action.

24. This was 'Der Kommende Tag' company's 'Clinical-Therapeutic Institute' that was in the process of being founded at the time. A medicines laboratory was attached to it, later called 'International laboratories'. Ultimately, like the Dornach medicines laboratory of the Futurum company, this merged with Weleda. More on this can be found in *Beiträge zur Rudolf Steiner Gesamtausgabe* (supplements to Rudolf Steiner's collected works), vol. 118/119, 'Rudolf Steiner und die Gründung der Weleda' ['Rudolf Steiner and the founding of Weleda'].

25. Shortly after the course ended, on 19 April 1921, a meeting must have taken place at Rudolf Steiner's house with the aim of drafting a document on the current state of medicines production. Alongside various physicians, the directors of the two laboratories, Dr Schmiedel for Dornach and Dr Kehler for Schwaebisch Gmünd, also attended. The basis for this meeting was probably a list compiled by Dr Schmiedel of 45 preparations, in turn based on an earlier

draft containing 39 preparations with handwritten notes by Rudolf Steiner. For more on this see *Beiträge zur Rudolf Steiner Gesamtausgabe* (supplements to Rudolf Steiner's collected works), vol. 118/119: 'Rudolf Steiner und die Gründung der Weleda' ['Rudolf Steiner and the founding of Weleda'].

26. CW 21, first published 1917.
27. Article by J.W. Hauer, in the periodical *Die Tat*, vol. 11 (February 1921), entitled 'Anthroposophy as path to the spirit'.
28. Jakob Wilhelm Hauer, 1881–1962, Indologist.
29. In earlier editions, for unknown reasons, this condition was cited as 'blood congestion below and ischaemia above'. The original shorthand transcript by Frau Finckh clearly records the words as printed here, which is also confirmed in a notebook entry (see supplement, p. 181).
30. Gustav Bunge, 1844–1920, physician, physiologist, professor in Basel, proponent of neovitalism.
31. See lecture 1 in *The Curative Eurythmy Course*, CW 315.

RUDOLF STEINER'S COLLECTED WORKS

The German Edition of Rudolf Steiner's Collected Works (the *Gesamtausgabe* [GA] published by Rudolf Steiner Verlag, Dornach, Switzerland) presently runs to 354 titles, organized either by type of work (written or spoken), chronology, audience (public or other), or subject (education, art, etc.). For ease of comparison, the Collected Works in English [CW] follows the German organization exactly. A complete listing of the CWs follows with literal translations of the German titles. Other than in the case of the books published in his lifetime, titles were rarely given by Rudolf Steiner himself, and were often provided by the editors of the German editions. The titles in English are not necessarily the same as the German; and, indeed, over the past seventy-five years have frequently been different, with the same book sometimes appearing under different titles.

For ease of identification and to avoid confusion, we suggest that readers looking for a title should do so by CW number. Because the work of creating the Collected Works of Rudolf Steiner is an ongoing process, with new titles being published every year, we have not indicated in this listing which books are presently available. To find out what titles in the Collected Works are currently in print, please check our website at www.rudolfsteinerpress.com (or www.steinerbooks.org for US readers).

Written Work

CW 1	Goethe: Natural-Scientific Writings, Introduction, with Footnotes and Explanations in the text by Rudolf Steiner
CW 2	Outlines of an Epistemology of the Goethean World View, with Special Consideration of Schiller
CW 3	Truth and Science
CW 4	The Philosophy of Freedom
CW 4a	Documents to 'The Philosophy of Freedom'
CW 5	Friedrich Nietzsche, A Fighter against His Own Time
CW 6	Goethe's Worldview
CW 6a	Now in CW 30
CW 7	Mysticism at the Dawn of Modern Spiritual Life and Its Relationship with Modern Worldviews
CW 8	Christianity as Mystical Fact and the Mysteries of Antiquity
CW 9	Theosophy: An Introduction into Supersensible World Knowledge and Human Purpose
CW 10	How Does One Attain Knowledge of Higher Worlds?
CW 11	From the Akasha-Chronicle

Public Lectures

Lectures to the Members of the Anthroposophical Society

206 * ILLNESS AND THERAPY

<table>
<tr><td>CW 150</td><td>The World of the Spirit and Its Extension into Physical Existence; The Influence of the Dead in the World of the Living</td></tr>
<tr><td>CW 151</td><td>Human Thought and Cosmic Thought</td></tr>
<tr><td>CW 152</td><td>Preliminary Stages to the Mystery of Golgotha</td></tr>
<tr><td>CW 153</td><td>The Inner Being of the Human Being and Life Between Death and New Birth</td></tr>
<tr><td>CW 154</td><td>How does One Gain an Understanding of the Spiritual World? The Flowing in of Spiritual Impulses from out of the World of the Deceased</td></tr>
<tr><td>CW 155</td><td>Christ and the Human Soul. Concerning the Meaning of Life. Theosophical Morality. Anthroposophy and Christianity</td></tr>
<tr><td>CW 156</td><td>Occult Reading and Occult Hearing</td></tr>
<tr><td>CW 157</td><td>Human Destinies and the Destiny of Peoples</td></tr>
<tr><td>CW 157a</td><td>The Formation of Destiny and the Life after Death</td></tr>
<tr><td>CW 158</td><td>The Connection Between the Human Being and the Elemental World. Kalevala—Olaf Asteson—The Russian People—The World as the Result of the Influences of Equilibrium</td></tr>
<tr><td>CW 159</td><td>The Mystery of Death. The Nature and Significance of Middle Europe and the European Folk Spirits</td></tr>
<tr><td>CW 160</td><td>In CW 159</td></tr>
<tr><td>CW 161</td><td>Paths of Spiritual Knowledge and the Renewal of the Artistic Worldview</td></tr>
<tr><td>CW 162</td><td>Questions of Art and Life in Light of Spiritual Science</td></tr>
<tr><td>CW 163</td><td>Coincidence, Necessity and Providence. Imaginative Knowledge and the Processes after Death</td></tr>
<tr><td>CW 164</td><td>The Value of Thinking for a Knowledge That Satisfies the Human Being. The Relationship of Spiritual Science to Natural Science</td></tr>
<tr><td>CW 165</td><td>The Spiritual Unification of Humanity through the Christ-Impulse</td></tr>
<tr><td>CW 166</td><td>Necessity and Freedom in the Events of the World and in Human Action</td></tr>
<tr><td>CW 167</td><td>The Present and the Past in the Human Spirit</td></tr>
<tr><td>CW 168</td><td>The Connection between the Living and the Dead</td></tr>
<tr><td>CW 169</td><td>World-being and Selfhood</td></tr>
<tr><td>CW 170</td><td>The Riddle of the Human Being. The Spiritual Background of Human History. Cosmic and Human History, Vol. 1</td></tr>
<tr><td>CW 171</td><td>Inner Development-Impulses of Humanity. Goethe and the Crisis of the 19th Century. Cosmic and Human History, Vol. 2</td></tr>
<tr><td>CW 172</td><td>The Karma of the Vocation of the Human Being in Connection with Goethe's Life. Cosmic and Human History, Vol. 3</td></tr>
<tr><td>CW 173</td><td>Contemporary-Historical Considerations: The Karma of Untruthfulness, Part One. Cosmic and Human History, Vol. 4</td></tr>
<tr><td>CW 174</td><td>Contemporary-Historical Considerations: The Karma of Untruthfulness, Part Two. Cosmic and Human History, Vol. 5</td></tr>
<tr><td>CW 174a</td><td>Middle Europe between East and West. Cosmic and Human History, Vol. 6</td></tr>
<tr><td>CW 174b</td><td>The Spiritual Background of the First World War. Cosmic and Human History, Vol. 7</td></tr>
</table>

CW 200   The New Spirituality and the Christ-Experience of the 20th Century
CW 201   The Correspondences Between Microcosm and Macrocosm. The Human Being—A Hieroglyph of the Universe. The Human Being in Relationship with the Cosmos: 1
CW 202   The Bridge between the World-Spirituality and the Physical Aspect of the Human Being. The Search for the New Isis, the Divine Sophia. The Human Being in Relationship with the Cosmos: 2
CW 203   The Responsibility of Human Beings for the Development of the World through their Spiritual Connection with the Planet Earth and the World of the Stars. The Human Being in Relationship with the Cosmos: 3
CW 204   Perspectives of the Development of Humanity. The Materialistic Knowledge-Impulse and the Task of Anthroposophy. The Human Being in Relationship with the Cosmos: 4
CW 205   Human Development, World-Soul, and World-Spirit. Part One: The Human Being as a Being of Body and Soul in Relationship to the World. The Human Being in Relationship with the Cosmos: 5
CW 206   Human Development, World-Soul, and World-Spirit. Part Two: The Human Being as a Spiritual Being in the Process of Historical Development. The Human Being in Relationship with the Cosmos: 6
CW 207   Anthroposophy as Cosmosophy. Part One: Characteristic Features of the Human Being in the Earthly and the Cosmic Realms. The Human Being in Relationship with the Cosmos: 7
CW 208   Anthroposophy as Cosmosophy. Part Two: The Forming of the Human Being as the Result of Cosmic Influence. The Human Being in Relationship with the Cosmos: 8
CW 209   Nordic and Central European Spiritual Impulses. The Festival of the Appearance of Christ. The Human Being in Relationship with the Cosmos: 9
CW 210   Old and New Methods of Initiation. Drama and Poetry in the Change of Consciousness in the Modern Age
CW 211   The Sun Mystery and the Mystery of Death and Resurrection. Exoteric and Esoteric Christianity
CW 212   Human Soul Life and Spiritual Striving in Connection with World and Earth Development
CW 213   Human Questions and World Answers
CW 214   The Mystery of the Trinity: The Human Being in Relationship with the Spiritual World in the Course of Time
CW 215   Philosophy, Cosmology, and Religion in Anthroposophy
CW 216   The Fundamental Impulses of the World-Historical Development of Humanity
CW 217   Spiritually Active Forces in the Coexistence of the Older and Younger Generations. Pedagogical Course for Youth

CW 240 — Esoteric Observations of Karmic Relationships in 6 Volumes, Vol. 6

CW 243 — The Consciousness of the Initiate

CW 245 — Instructions for an Esoteric Schooling

CW 250 — The Building-Up of the Anthroposophical Society. From the Beginning to the Outbreak of the First World War

CW 251 — The History of the Goetheanum Building-Association

CW 252 — Life in the Anthroposophical Society from the First World War to the Burning of the First Goetheanum

CW 253 — The Problems of Living Together in the Anthroposophical Society. On the Dornach Crisis of 1915. With Highlights on Swedenborg's Clairvoyance, the Views of Freudian Psychoanalysts, and the Concept of Love in Relation to Mysticism

CW 254 — The Occult Movement in the 19th Century and Its Relationship to World Culture. Significant Points from the Exoteric Cultural Life around the Middle of the 19th Century

CW 255 — Rudolf Steiner during the First World War

CW 255a — Anthroposophy and the Reformation of Society. On the History of the Threefold Movement

CW 255b — Anthroposophy and Its Opponents, 1919–1921

CW 256 — How Can the Anthroposophical Movement Be Financed?

CW 256a — Futurum, Inc. / International Laboratories, Inc.

CW 256b — The Coming Day, Inc.

CW 257 — Anthroposophical Community-Building

CW 258 — The History of and Conditions for the Anthroposophical Movement in Relationship to the Anthroposophical Society. A Stimulus to Self-Contemplation

CW 259 — The Year of Destiny 1923 in the History of the Anthroposophical Society. From the Burning of the Goetheanum to the Christmas Conference

CW 260 — The Christmas Conference for the Founding of the General Anthroposophical Society

CW 260a — The Constitution of the General Anthroposophical Society and the School for Spiritual Science. The Rebuilding of the Goetheanum

CW 261 — Our Dead. Addresses, Words of Remembrance, and Meditative Verses, 1906–1924

CW 262 — Rudolf Steiner and Marie Steiner-von Sivers: Correspondence and Documents, 1901–1925

CW 263/1 — Rudolf Steiner and Edith Maryon: Correspondence: Letters, Verses, Sketches, 1912–1924

CW 264 — On the History and the Contents of the First Section of the Esoteric School from 1904 to 1914. Letters, Newsletters, Documents, Lectures

CW 265 — On the History and from the Contents of the Ritual-Knowledge Section of the Esoteric School from 1904 to 1914. Documents, and Lectures from the Years 1906 to 1914, as Well as on New Approaches to Ritual-Knowledge Work in the Years 1921–1924

SIGNIFICANT EVENTS IN THE LIFE OF
RUDOLF STEINER

1829:   June 23: birth of Johann Steiner (1829–1910)—Rudolf Steiner's
         father—in Geras, Lower Austria.
1834:   May 8: birth of Franciska Blie (1834–1918)—Rudolf Steiner's mother—
         in Horn, Lower Austria. 'My father and mother were both children of the
         glorious Lower Austrian forest district north of the Danube.'
1860:   May 16: marriage of Johann Steiner and Franciska Blie.
1861:   February 25: birth of *Rudolf Joseph Lorenz Steiner* in Kraljevec, Croatia,
         near the border with Hungary, where Johann Steiner works as a tele-
         grapher for the South Austria Railroad. Rudolf Steiner is baptized two
         days later, February 27, the date usually given as his birthday.
1862:   Summer: the family moves to Mödling, Lower Austria.
1863:   The family moves to Pottschach, Lower Austria, near the Styrian border,
         where Johann Steiner becomes stationmaster. 'The view stretched to the
         mountains ... majestic peaks in the distance and the sweet charm of
         nature in the immediate surroundings.'
1864:   November 15: birth of Rudolf Steiner's sister, Leopoldine (d. November
         1, 1927). She will become a seamstress and live with her parents for the
         rest of her life.
1866:   July 28: birth of Rudolf Steiner's deaf-mute brother, Gustav (d. May 1,
         1941).
1867:   Rudolf Steiner enters the village school. Following a disagreement
         between his father and the schoolmaster, whose wife falsely accused the
         boy of causing a commotion, Rudolf Steiner is taken out of school and
         taught at home.
1868:   A critical experience. Unknown to the family, an aunt dies in a distant
         town. Sitting in the station waiting room, Rudolf Steiner sees her 'form,'
         which speaks to him, asking for help. 'Beginning with this experience, a
         new soul life began in the boy, one in which not only the outer trees and
         mountains spoke to him, but also the worlds that lay behind them. From
         this moment on, the boy began to live with the spirits of nature ...'
1869:   The family moves to the peaceful, rural village of Neudorfl, near Wiener-
         Neustadt in present-day Austria. Rudolf Steiner attends the village
         school. Because of the 'unorthodoxy' of his writing and spelling, he has to
         do 'extra lessons.'
1870:   Through a book lent to him by his tutor, he discovers geometry: 'To
         grasp something purely in the spirit brought me inner happiness. I know
         that I first learned happiness through geometry.' The same tutor allows

him to draw, while other students still struggle with their reading and writing. 'An artistic element' thus enters his education.

1871:   Though his parents are not religious, Rudolf Steiner becomes a 'church child,' a favorite of the priest, who was 'an exceptional character.' 'Up to the age of ten or eleven, among those I came to know, he was far and away the most significant.' Among other things, he introduces Steiner to Copernican, heliocentric cosmology. As an altar boy, Rudolf Steiner serves at Masses, funerals, and Corpus Christi processions. At year's end, after an incident in which he escapes a thrashing, his father forbids him to go to church.

1872:   Rudolf Steiner transfers to grammar school in Wiener-Neustadt, a five-mile walk from home, which must be done in all weathers.

1873–75: Through his teachers and on his own, Rudolf Steiner has many wonderful experiences with science and mathematics. Outside school, he teaches himself analytic geometry, trigonometry, differential equations, and calculus.

1876:   Rudolf Steiner begins tutoring other students. He learns bookbinding from his father. He also teaches himself stenography.

1877:   Rudolf Steiner discovers Kant's *Critique of Pure Reason*, which he reads and rereads. He also discovers and reads von Rotteck's *World History*.

1878:   He studies extensively in contemporary psychology and philosophy.

1879:   Rudolf Steiner graduates from high school with honors. His father is transferred to Inzersdorf, near Vienna. He uses his first visit to Vienna 'to purchase a great number of philosophy books'—Kant, Fichte, Schelling, and Hegel, as well as numerous histories of philosophy. His aim: to find a path from the 'I' to nature.

October 1879–1883: Rudolf Steiner attends the Technical College in Vienna—to study mathematics, chemistry, physics, mineralogy, botany, zoology, biology, geology, and mechanics—with a scholarship. He also attends lectures in history and literature, while avidly reading philosophy on his own. His two favorite professors are Karl Julius Schröer (German language and literature) and Edmund Reitlinger (physics). He also audits lectures by Robert Zimmerman on aesthetics and Franz Brentano on philosophy. During this year he begins his friendship with Moritz Zitter (1861–1921), who will help support him financially when he is in Berlin.

1880:   Rudolf Steiner attends lectures on Schiller and Goethe by Karl Julius Schröer, who becomes his mentor. Also 'through a remarkable combination of circumstances,' he meets Felix Koguzki, a 'herb gatherer' and healer, who could 'see deeply into the secrets of nature.' Rudolf Steiner will meet and study with this 'emissary of the Master' throughout his time in Vienna.

1881:   January: '... I didn't sleep a wink. I was busy with philosophical problems until about 12:30 a.m. Then, finally, I threw myself down on my couch. All my striving during the previous year had been to research whether the following statement by Schelling was true or not: *Within everyone dwells a secret, marvelous capacity to draw back from the stream of time—out of the self clothed in all that comes to us from outside—into our innermost being and there, in the immutable form of the Eternal, to look into ourselves.* I believe, and I am still quite certain of it, that I discovered this capacity in myself; I had long had an inkling of it. Now the whole of idealist philosophy stood before me in modified form. What's a sleepless night compared to that!'

Rudolf Steiner begins communicating with leading thinkers of the day, who send him books in return, which he reads eagerly.

July: 'I am not one of those who dives into the day like an animal in human form. I pursue a quite specific goal, an idealistic aim—knowledge of the truth! This cannot be done offhandedly. It requires the greatest striving in the world, free of all egotism, and equally of all resignation.'

August: Steiner puts down on paper for the first time thoughts for a 'Philosophy of Freedom.' 'The striving for the absolute: this human yearning is freedom.' He also seeks to outline a 'peasant philosophy,' describing what the worldview of a 'peasant'—one who lives close to the earth and the old ways—really is.

1881–1882: Felix Koguzki, the herb gatherer, reveals himself to be the envoy of another, higher initiatory personality, who instructs Rudolf Steiner to penetrate Fichte's philosophy and to master modern scientific thinking as a preparation for right entry into the spirit. This 'Master' also teaches him the double (evolutionary and involutionary) nature of time.

1882: Through the offices of Karl Julius Schröer, Rudolf Steiner is asked by Joseph Kurschner to edit Goethe's scientific works for the *Deutschen National-Literatur* edition. He writes 'A Possible Critique of Atomistic Concepts' and sends it to Friedrich Theodore Vischer.

1883: Rudolf Steiner completes his college studies and begins work on the Goethe project.

1884: First volume of Goethe's *Scientific Writings* (CW 1) appears (March). He lectures on Goethe and Lessing, and Goethe's approach to science. In July, he enters the household of Ladislaus and Pauline Specht as tutor to the four Specht boys. He will live there until 1890. At this time, he meets Josef Breuer (1842–1925), the coauthor with Sigmund Freud of *Studies in Hysteria*, who is the Specht family doctor.

1885: While continuing to edit Goethe's writings, Rudolf Steiner reads deeply in contemporary philosophy (Edouard von Hartmann, Johannes Volkelt, and Richard Wahle, among others).

1886: May: Rudolf Steiner sends Kurschner the manuscript of *Outlines of Goethe's Theory of Knowledge* (CW 2), which appears in October, and which he sends out widely. He also meets the poet Marie Eugenie Delle Grazie and writes 'Nature and Our Ideals' for her. He attends her salon, where he meets many priests, theologians, and philosophers, who will become his friends. Meanwhile, the director of the Goethe Archive in Weimar requests his collaboration with the *Sophien* edition of Goethe's works, particularly the writings on color.

1887: At the beginning of the year, Rudolf Steiner is very sick. As the year progresses and his health improves, he becomes increasingly 'a man of letters,' lecturing, writing essays, and taking part in Austrian cultural life. In August–September, the second volume of Goethe's *Scientific Writings* appears.

1888: January–July: Rudolf Steiner assumes editorship of the 'German Weekly' (*Deutsche Wochenschrift*). He begins lecturing more intensively, giving, for example, a lecture titled 'Goethe as Father of a New Aesthetics.' He meets and becomes soul friends with Friedrich Eckstein (1861–1939), a vegetarian, philosopher of symbolism, alchemist, and musician, who will introduce him to various spiritual currents (including Theosophy) and with whom he will meditate and interpret esoteric and alchemical texts.

1889: Rudolf Steiner first reads Nietzsche (*Beyond Good and Evil*). He encounters Theosophy again and learns of Madame Blavatsky in the Theosophical circle around Marie Lang (1858–1934). Here he also meets well-known figures of Austrian life, as well as esoteric figures like the occultist Franz Hartman and Karl Leinigen-Billigen (translator of C.G. Harrison's *The Transcendental Universe*). During this period, Steiner first reads A.P. Sinnett's *Esoteric Buddhism* and Mabel Collins's *Light on the Path*. He also begins traveling, visiting Budapest, Weimar, and Berlin (where he meets philosopher Edouard von Hartmann).

1890: Rudolf Steiner finishes volume 3 of Goethe's scientific writings. He begins his doctoral dissertation, which will become *Truth and Science* (CW 3). He also meets the poet and feminist Rosa Mayreder (1858–1938), with whom he can exchange his most intimate thoughts. In September, Rudolf Steiner moves to Weimar to work in the Goethe-Schiller Archive.

1891: Volume 3 of the Kurschner edition of Goethe appears. Meanwhile, Rudolf Steiner edits Goethe's studies in mineralogy and scientific writings for the *Sophien* edition. He meets Ludwig Laistner of the Cotta Publishing Company, who asks for a book on the basic question of metaphysics. From this will result, ultimately, *The Philosophy of Freedom* (CW 4), which will be published not by Cotta but by Emil Felber. In October, Rudolf Steiner takes the oral exam for a doctorate in philosophy, mathematics, and mechanics at Rostock University, receiving his doctorate on the twenty-sixth. In November, he gives his first lecture on Goethe's 'Fairy Tale' in Vienna.

1892: Rudolf Steiner continues work at the Goethe-Schiller Archive and on his *Philosophy of Freedom*. *Truth and Science*, his doctoral dissertation, is published. Steiner undertakes to write introductions to books on Schopenhauer and Jean Paul for Cotta. At year's end, he finds lodging with Anna Eunike, née Schulz (1853–1911), a widow with four daughters and a son. He also develops a friendship with Otto Erich Hartleben (1864–1905) with whom he shares literary interests.

1893: Rudolf Steiner begins his habit of producing many reviews and articles. In March, he gives a lecture titled 'Hypnotism, with Reference to Spiritism.' In September, volume 4 of the Kurschner edition is completed. In November, *The Philosophy of Freedom* appears. This year, too, he meets John Henry Mackay (1864–1933), the anarchist, and Max Stirner, a scholar and biographer.

1894: Rudolf Steiner meets Elisabeth Förster Nietzsche, the philosopher's sister, and begins to read Nietzsche in earnest, beginning with the as yet unpublished *Antichrist*. He also meets Ernst Haeckel (1834–1919). In the fall, he begins to write *Nietzsche, A Fighter against His Time* (CW 5).

1895:   May, *Nietzsche, A Fighter against His Time* appears.

1896:   January 22: Rudolf Steiner sees Friedrich Nietzsche for the first and only time. Moves between the Nietzsche and the Goethe-Schiller Archives, where he completes his work before year's end. He falls out with Elisabeth Förster Nietzsche, thus ending his association with the Nietzsche Archive.

1897:   Rudolf Steiner finishes the manuscript of *Goethe's Worldview* (CW 6). He moves to Berlin with Anna Eunike and begins editorship of the *Magazin für Literatur*. From now on, Steiner will write countless reviews, literary and philosophical articles, and so on. He begins lecturing at the 'Free Literary Society.' In September, he attends the Zionist Congress in Basel. He sides with Dreyfus in the Dreyfus affair.

1898:   Rudolf Steiner is very active as an editor in the political, artistic, and theatrical life of Berlin. He becomes friendly with John Henry Mackay and poet Ludwig Jacobowski (1868–1900). He joins Jacobowski's circle of writers, artists, and scientists—'The Coming Ones' (*Die Kommenden*)— and contributes lectures to the group until 1903. He also lectures at the 'League for College Pedagogy.' He writes an article for Goethe's sesquicentennial, 'Goethe's Secret Revelation,' on the 'Fairy Tale of the Green Snake and the Beautiful Lily.'

1898–99: 'This was a trying time for my soul as I looked at Christianity. . . . I was able to progress only by contemplating, by means of spiritual perception, the evolution of Christianity. . . . Conscious knowledge of real Christianity began to dawn in me around the turn of the century. This seed continued to develop. My soul trial occurred shortly before the beginning of the twentieth century. It was decisive for my soul's development that I stood spiritually before the Mystery of Golgotha in a deep and solemn celebration of knowledge.'

1899:   Rudolf Steiner begins teaching and giving lectures and lecture cycles at the Workers' College, founded by Wilhelm Liebknecht (1826–1900). He will continue to do so until 1904. Writes: *Literature and Spiritual Life in the Nineteenth Century; Individualism in Philosophy; Haeckel and His Opponents; Poetry in the Present;* and begins what will become (fifteen years later) *The Riddles of Philosophy* (CW 18). He also meets many artists and writers, including Käthe Kollwitz, Stefan Zweig, and Rainer Maria Rilke. On October 31, he marries Anna Eunike.

1900:   'I thought that the turn of the century must bring humanity a new light. It seemed to me that the separation of human thinking and willing from the spirit had peaked. A turn or reversal of direction in human evolution seemed to me a necessity.' Rudolf Steiner finishes *World and Life Views in the Nineteenth Century* (the second part of what will become *The Riddles of Philosophy*) and dedicates it to Ernst Haeckel. It is published in March. He continues lecturing at *Die Kommenden*, whose leadership he assumes after the death of Jacobowski. Also, he gives the Gutenberg Jubilee lecture before 7,000 typesetters and printers. In September, Rudolf Steiner is invited by Count and Countess Brockdorff to lecture in the Theosophical Library. His first lecture is on Nietzsche. His second lecture is titled 'Goethe's Secret Revelation.' October 6, he begins a lecture cycle on the mystics that will become *Mystics after Modernism* (CW 7). November-December: 'Marie von Sivers appears in the audience....' Also in November, Steiner gives his first lecture at the Giordano Bruno Bund (where he will continue to lecture until May, 1905). He speaks on Bruno and modern Rome, focusing on the importance of the philosophy of Thomas Aquinas as monism.

1901:   In continual financial straits, Rudolf Steiner's early friends Moritz Zitter and Rosa Mayreder help support him. In October, he begins the lecture cycle *Christianity as Mystical Fact* (CW 8) at the Theosophical Library. In November, he gives his first 'Theosophical lecture' on Goethe's 'Fairy Tale' in Hamburg at the invitation of Wilhelm Hubbe-Schleiden. He also attends a gathering to celebrate the founding of the Theosophical Society at Count and Countess Brockdorff's. He gives a lecture cycle, 'From Buddha to Christ,' for the circle of the *Kommenden*. November 17, Marie von Sivers asks Rudolf Steiner if Theosophy needs a Western-Christian spiritual movement (to complement Theosophy's Eastern emphasis). 'The question was posed. Now, following spiritual laws, I could begin to give an answer....' In December, Rudolf Steiner writes his first article for a Theosophical publication. At year's end, the Brockdorffs and possibly Wilhelm Hubbe-Schleiden ask Rudolf Steiner to join the Theosophical Society and undertake the leadership of the German section. Rudolf Steiner agrees, on the condition that Marie von Sivers (then in Italy) work with him.

1902:   Beginning in January, Rudolf Steiner attends the opening of the Workers' School in Spandau with Rosa Luxemberg (1870–1919). January 17, Rudolf Steiner joins the Theosophical Society. In April, he is asked to become general secretary of the German Section of the Theosophical Society, and works on preparations for its founding. In July, he visits London for a Theosophical congress. He meets Bertram Keightly, G.R.S. Mead, A.P. Sinnett, and Annie Besant, among others. In September, *Christianity as Mystical Fact* appears. In October, Rudolf Steiner gives his first public lecture on Theosophy ('Monism and Theosophy') to about three hundred people at the Giordano Bruno Bund. On October 19–21, the German Section of the Theosophical Society has its first meeting; Rudolf Steiner is the general secretary, and Annie Besant attends. Steiner lectures on practical karma studies. On October 23, Annie Besant inducts Rudolf Steiner into the Esoteric School of the Theosophical Society. On October 25, Steiner begins a weekly series of lectures: 'The Field of Theosophy.' During this year, Rudolf Steiner also first meets Ita Wegman (1876–1943), who will become his close collaborator in his final years.

1903:   Rudolf Steiner holds about 300 lectures and seminars. In May, the first issue of the periodical *Luzifer* appears. In June, Rudolf Steiner visits

London for the first meeting of the Federation of the European Sections of the Theosophical Society, where he meets Colonel Olcott. He begins to write *Theosophy* (CW 9).

1904: Rudolf Steiner continues lecturing at the Workers' College and elsewhere (about 90 lectures), while lecturing intensively all over Germany among Theosophists (about 140 lectures). In February, he meets Carl Unger (1878–1929), who will become a member of the board of the Anthroposophical Society (1913). In March, he meets Michael Bauer (1871–1929), a Christian mystic, who will also be on the board. In May, *Theosophy* appears, with the dedication: 'To the spirit of Giordano Bruno.' Rudolf Steiner and Marie von Sivers visit London for meetings with Annie Besant. June: Rudolf Steiner and Marie von Sivers attend the meeting of the Federation of European Sections of the Theosophical Society in Amsterdam. In July, Steiner begins the articles in *Luzifer-Gnosis* that will become *How to Know Higher Worlds* (CW 10) and *Cosmic Memory* (CW 11). In September, Annie Besant visits Germany. In December, Steiner lectures on Freemasonry. He mentions the High Grade Masonry derived from John Yarker and represented by Theodore Reuss and Karl Kellner as a blank slate 'into which a good image could be placed.'

1905: This year, Steiner ends his non-Theosophical lecturing activity. Supported by Marie von Sivers, his Theosophical lecturing—both in public and in the Theosophical Society—increases significantly: 'The German Theosophical Movement is of exceptional importance.' Steiner recommends reading, among others, Fichte, Jacob Boehme, and Angelus Silesius. He begins to introduce Christian themes into Theosophy. He also begins to work with doctors (Felix Peipers and Ludwig Noll). In July, he is in London for the Federation of European Sections, where he attends a lecture by Annie Besant: 'I have seldom seen Mrs. Besant speak in so inward and heartfelt a manner....' 'Through Mrs. Besant I have found the way to H.P. Blavatsky.' September to October, he gives a course of thirty-one lectures for a small group of esoteric students. In October, the annual meeting of the German Section of the Theosophical Society, which still remains very small, takes place. Rudolf Steiner reports membership has risen from 121 to 377 members. In November, seeking to establish esoteric 'continuity,' Rudolf Steiner and Marie von Sivers participate in a 'Memphis-Misraim' Masonic ceremony. They pay forty-five marks for membership. 'Yesterday, you saw how little remains of former esoteric institutions.' 'We are dealing only with a "framework"... for the present, nothing lies behind it. The occult powers have completely withdrawn.'

1906: Expansion of Theosophical work. Rudolf Steiner gives about 245 lectures, only 44 of which take place in Berlin. Cycles are given in Paris, Leipzig, Stuttgart, and Munich. Esoteric work also intensifies. Rudolf Steiner begins writing *An Outline of Esoteric Science* (CW 13). In January, Rudolf Steiner receives permission (a patent) from the Great Orient of the Scottish A & A Thirty-Three Degree Rite of the Order of the Ancient

Freemasons of the Memphis-Misraim Rite to direct a chapter under the name 'Mystica Aeterna.' This will become the 'Cognitive-Ritual Section' (also called 'Misraim Service') of the Esoteric School. (See: *Freemasonry and Ritual Work: The Misraim Service*, CW 265). During this time, Steiner also meets Albert Schweitzer. In May, he is in Paris, where he visits Edouard Schuré. Many Russians attend his lectures (including Konstantin Balmont, Dimitri Mereszkovski, Zinaida Hippius, and Maximilian Woloshin). He attends the General Meeting of the European Federation of the Theosophical Society, at which Col. Olcott is present for the last time. He spends the year's end in Venice and Rome, where he writes and works on his translation of H.P. Blavatsky's *Key to Theosophy*.

1907:   Further expansion of the German Theosophical Movement according to the Rosicrucian directive to 'introduce spirit into the world'—in education, in social questions, in art, and in science. In February, Col. Olcott dies in Adyar. Before he dies, Olcott indicates that 'the Masters' wish Annie Besant to succeed him: much politicking ensues. Rudolf Steiner supports Besant's candidacy. April-May: preparations for the Congress of the Federation of European Sections of the Theosophical Society—the great, watershed Whitsun 'Munich Congress,' attended by Annie Besant and others. Steiner decides to separate Eastern and Western (Christian-Rosicrucian) esoteric schools. He takes his esoteric school out of the Theosophical Society (Besant and Rudolf Steiner are 'in harmony' on this). Steiner makes his first lecture tours to Austria and Hungary. That summer, he is in Italy. In September, he visits Edouard Schuré, who will write the introduction to the French edition of *Christianity as Mystical Fact* in Barr, Alsace. Rudolf Steiner writes the autobiographical statement known as the 'Barr Document.' In *Luzifer-Gnosis*, 'The Education of the Child' appears.

1908:   The movement grows (membership: 1,150). Lecturing expands. Steiner makes his first extended lecture tour to Holland and Scandinavia, as well as visits to Naples and Sicily. Themes: St. John's Gospel, the Apocalypse, Egypt, science, philosophy, and logic. *Luzifer-Gnosis* ceases publication. In Berlin, Marie von Sivers (with Johanna Mücke (1864–1949) forms the *Philosophisch-Theosophisch* (after 1915 *Philosophisch-Anthroposophisch*) *Verlag* to publish Steiner's work. Steiner gives lecture cycles titled *The Gospel of St. John* (CW 103) and *The Apocalypse* (104).

1909:   *An Outline of Esoteric Science* appears. Lecturing and travel continues. Rudolf Steiner's spiritual research expands to include the polarity of Lucifer and Ahriman; the work of great individualities in history; the Maitreya Buddha and the Bodhisattvas; spiritual economy (CW 109); the work of the spiritual hierarchies in heaven and on earth (CW 110). He also deepens and intensifies his research into the Gospels, giving lectures on the Gospel of St. Luke (CW 114) with the first mention of two Jesus children. Meets and becomes friends with Christian Morgenstern (1871–1914). In April, he lays the foundation stone for the Malsch model—the building that will lead to the first Goetheanum. In May, the International Congress of the Federation of European Sections of the

Theosophical Society takes place in Budapest. Rudolf Steiner receives the Subba Row medal for *How to Know Higher Worlds*. During this time, Charles W. Leadbeater discovers Jiddu Krishnamurti (1895–1986) and proclaims him the future 'world teacher,' the bearer of the Maitreya Buddha and the 'reappearing Christ.' In October, Steiner delivers seminal lectures on 'anthroposophy,' which he will try, unsuccessfully, to rework over the next years into the unfinished work, *Anthroposophy (A Fragment)* (CW 45).

1910: New themes: *The Reappearance of Christ in the Etheric* (CW 118); *The Fifth Gospel; The Mission of Folk Souls* (CW 121); *Occult History* (CW 126); the evolving development of etheric cognitive capacities. Rudolf Steiner continues his Gospel research with *The Gospel of St. Matthew* (CW 123). In January, his father dies. In April, he takes a month-long trip to Italy, including Rome, Monte Cassino, and Sicily. He also visits Scandinavia again. July–August, he writes the first mystery drama, *The Portal of Initiation* (CW 14). In November, he gives 'psychosophy' lectures. In December, he submits 'On the Psychological Foundations and Epistemological Framework of Theosophy' to the International Philosophical Congress in Bologna.

1911: The crisis in the Theosophical Society deepens. In January, 'The Order of the Rising Sun,' which will soon become 'The Order of the Star in the East,' is founded for the coming world teacher, Krishnamurti. At the same time, Marie von Sivers, Rudolf Steiner's coworker, falls ill. Fewer lectures are given, but important new ground is broken. In Prague, in March, Steiner meets Franz Kafka (1883–1924) and Hugo Bergmann (1883-1975). In April, he delivers his paper to the Philosophical Congress. He writes the second mystery drama, *The Soul's Probation* (CW 14). Also, while Marie von Sivers is convalescing, Rudolf Steiner begins work on *Calendar 1912/1913*, which will contain the 'Calendar of the Soul' meditations. On March 19, Anna (Eunike) Steiner dies. In September, Rudolf Steiner visits Einsiedeln, birthplace of Paracelsus. In December, Friedrich Rittelmeyer, future founder of the Christian Community, meets Rudolf Steiner. The *Johannes-Bauverein*, the 'building committee,' which would lead to the first Goetheanum (first planned for Munich), is also founded, and a preliminary committee for the founding of an independent association is created that, in the following year, will become the Anthroposophical Society. Important lecture cycles include *Occult Physiology* (CW 128); *Wonders of the World* (CW 129); *From Jesus to Christ* (CW 131). Other themes: esoteric Christianity; Christian Rosenkreutz; the spiritual guidance of humanity; the sense world and the world of the spirit.

1912: Despite the ongoing, now increasing crisis in the Theosophical Society, much is accomplished: *Calendar 1912/1913* is published; eurythmy is created; both the third mystery drama, *The Guardian of the Threshold* (CW 14) and *A Way of Self-Knowledge* (CW 16) are written. New (or renewed) themes included life between death and rebirth and karma and reincarnation. Other lecture cycles: *Spiritual Beings in the Heavenly Bodies and in the Kingdoms of Nature* (CW 136); *The Human Being in the Light of Occultism, Theosophy, and Philosophy* (CW 137); *The Gospel of St. Mark* (CW 139); and *The Bhagavad Gita and the Epistles of Paul* (CW 142). On May 8, Rudolf Steiner celebrates White Lotus Day, H.P. Blavatsky's death day, which he had faithfully observed for the past decade, for the last time. In August, Rudolf Steiner suggests the 'independent association' be called the 'Anthroposophical Society.' In September, the first eurythmy course takes place. In October, Rudolf Steiner declines recognition of a Theosophical Society lodge dedicated to the Star of the East and decides to expel all Theosophical Society members belonging to the order. Also, with Marie von Sivers, he first visits Dornach, near Basel, Switzerland, and they stand on the hill where the Goetheanum will be built. In November, a Theosophical Society lodge is opened by direct mandate from Adyar (Annie Besant). In December, a meeting of the German section occurs at which it is decided that belonging to the Order of the Star of the East is incompatible with membership in the Theosophical Society. December 28: informal founding of the Anthroposophical Society in Berlin.

1913: Expulsion of the German section from the Theosophical Society. February 2–3: Foundation meeting of the Anthroposophical Society. Board members include: Marie von Sivers, Michael Bauer, and Carl Unger. September 20: Laying of the foundation stone for the *Johannes Bau* (Goetheanum) in Dornach. Building begins immediately. The third mystery drama, *The Soul's Awakening* (CW 14), is completed. Also: *The Threshold of the Spiritual World* (CW 147). Lecture cycles include: *The Bhagavad Gita and the Epistles of Paul* and *The Esoteric Meaning of the Bhagavad Gita* (CW 146), which the Russian philosopher Nikolai Berdyaev attends; *The Mysteries of the East and of Christianity* (CW 144); *The Effects of Esoteric Development* (CW 145); and *The Fifth Gospel* (CW 148). In May, Rudolf Steiner is in London and Paris, where anthroposophical work continues.

1914: Building continues on the *Johannes Bau* (Goetheanum) in Dornach, with artists and coworkers from seventeen nations. The general assembly of the Anthroposophical Society takes place. In May, Rudolf Steiner visits Paris, as well as Chartres Cathedral. June 28: assassination in Sarajevo ('Now the catastrophe has happened!'). August 1: War is declared. Rudolf Steiner returns to Germany from Dornach—he will travel back and forth. He writes the last chapter of *The Riddles of Philosophy*. Lecture cycles include: *Human and Cosmic Thought* (CW 151); *Inner Being of Humanity between Death and a New Birth* (CW 153); *Occult Reading and Occult Hearing* (CW 156). December 24: marriage of Rudolf Steiner and Marie von Sivers.

1915: Building continues. Life after death becomes a major theme, also art. Writes: *Thoughts during a Time of War* (CW 24). Lectures include: *The Secret of Death* (CW 159); *The Uniting of Humanity through the Christ Impulse* (CW 165).

1916: Rudolf Steiner begins work with Edith Maryon (1872–1924) on the sculpture 'The Representative of Humanity' ('The Group'—Christ, Lucifer, and Ahriman). He also works with the alchemist Alexander von Bernus on the quarterly *Das Reich*. He writes *The Riddle of Humanity* (CW 20). Lectures include: *Necessity and Freedom in World History and Human Action* (CW 166); *Past and Present in the Human Spirit* (CW 167); *The Karma of Vocation* (CW 172); *The Karma of Untruthfulness* (CW 173).

1917: Russian Revolution. The U.S. enters the war. Building continues. Rudolf Steiner delineates the idea of the 'threefold nature of the human being' (in a public lecture March 15) and the 'threefold nature of the social organism' (hammered out in May-June with the help of Otto von Lerchenfeld and Ludwig Polzer-Hoditz in the form of two documents titled *Memoranda*, which were distributed in high places). August–September: Rudolf Steiner writes *The Riddles of the Soul* (CW 20). Also: commentary on 'The Chemical Wedding of Christian Rosenkreutz' for Alexander Bernus (*Das Reich*). Lectures include: *The Karma of Materialism* (CW 176); *The Spiritual Background of the Outer World: The Fall of the Spirits of Darkness* (CW 177).

1918: March 18: peace treaty of Brest-Litovsk—'Now everything will truly enter chaos! What is needed is cultural renewal.' June: Rudolf Steiner visits Karlstein (Grail) Castle outside Prague. Lecture cycle: *From Symptom to Reality in Modern History* (CW 185). In mid-November, Emil Molt, of the Waldorf-Astoria Cigarette Company, has the idea of founding a school for his workers' children.

1919: Focus on the threefold social organism: tireless travel, countless lectures, meetings, and publications. At the same time, a new public stage of Anthroposophy emerges as cultural renewal begins. The coming years will see initiatives in pedagogy, medicine, pharmacology, and agriculture. January 27: threefold meeting: ' We must first of all, with the money we have, found free schools that can bring people what they need.' February: first public eurythmy performance in Zurich. Also: 'Appeal to the German People' (CW 24), circulated March 6 as a newspaper insert. In April, *Towards Social Renewal* (CW 23) appears— 'perhaps the most widely read of all books on politics appearing since the war.' Rudolf Steiner is asked to undertake the 'direction and leadership' of the school founded by the Waldorf-Astoria Company. Rudolf Steiner begins to talk about the 'renewal' of education. May 30: a building is selected and purchased for the future Waldorf School. August–September, Rudolf Steiner gives a lecture course for Waldorf teachers, *The Foundations of Human Experience (Study of Man)* (CW 293). September 7: Opening of the first Waldorf School. December (into January): first science course, the *Light Course* (CW 320).

1920: The Waldorf School flourishes. New threefold initiatives. Founding of limited companies *Der Kommende Tag* and *Futurum A.G.* to infuse spiritual values into the economic realm. Rudolf Steiner also focuses on the sciences. Lectures: *Introducing Anthroposophical Medicine* (CW 312); *The Warmth Course* (CW 321); *The Boundaries of Natural Science* (CW 322); *The Redemption of Thinking* (CW 74). February: Johannes Werner

Klein—later a cofounder of the Christian Community—asks Rudolf Steiner about the possibility of a 'religious renewal,' a 'Johannine church.' In March, Rudolf Steiner gives the first course for doctors and medical students. In April, a divinity student asks Rudolf Steiner a second time about the possibility of religious renewal. September 27–October 16: anthroposophical 'university course.' December: lectures titled *The Search for the New Isis* (CW 202).

1921:   Rudolf Steiner continues his intensive work on cultural renewal, including the uphill battle for the threefold social order. 'University' arts, scientific, theological, and medical courses include: *The Astronomy Course* (CW 323); *Observation, Mathematics, and Scientific Experiment* (CW 324); the *Second Medical Course* (CW 313); *Color*. In June and September-October, Rudolf Steiner also gives the first two 'priests' courses' (CW 342 and 343). The 'youth movement' gains momentum. Magazines are founded: *Die Drei* (January), and—under the editorship of Albert Steffen (1884–1963)—the weekly, *Das Goetheanum* (August). In February–March, Rudolf Steiner takes his first trip outside Germany since the war (Holland). On April 7, Steiner receives a letter regarding 'religious renewal,' and May 22–23, he agrees to address the question in a practical way. In June, the Klinical-Therapeutic Institute opens in Arlesheim under the direction of Dr. Ita Wegman. In August, the Chemical-Pharmaceutical Laboratory opens in Arlesheim (Oskar Schmiedel and Ita Wegman are directors). The Clinical Therapeutic Institute is inaugurated in Stuttgart (Dr. Ludwig Noll is director); also the Research Laboratory in Dornach (Ehrenfried Pfeiffer and Gunther Wachsmuth are directors). In November–December, Rudolf Steiner visits Norway.

1922:   The first half of the year involves very active public lecturing (thousands attend); in the second half, Rudolf Steiner begins to withdraw and turn toward the Society—'The Society is asleep.' It is 'too weak' to do what is asked of it. The businesses—*Der Kommende Tag* and *Futurum A.G.*—fail. In January, with the help of an agent, Steiner undertakes a twelve-city German lecture tour, accompanied by eurythmy performances. In two weeks he speaks to more than 2,000 people. In April, he gives a 'university course' in The Hague. He also visits England. In June, he is in Vienna for the East–West Congress. In August–September, he is back in England for the Oxford Conference on Education. Returning to Dornach, he gives the lectures *Philosophy, Cosmology, and Religion* (CW 215), and gives the third priests' course (CW 344). On September 16, The Christian Community is founded. In October–November, Steiner is in Holland and England. He also speaks to the youth: *The Youth Course* (CW 217). In December, Steiner gives lectures titled *The Origins of Natural Science* (CW 326), and *Humanity and the World of Stars: The Spiritual Communion of Humanity* (CW 219). December 31: Fire at the Goetheanum, which is destroyed.

1923:   Despite the fire, Rudolf Steiner continues his work unabated. A very hard year. Internal dispersion, dissension, and apathy abound. There is conflict—between old and new visions—within the Society. A wake-up call is needed, and Rudolf Steiner responds with renewed lecturing vitality. His focus: the spiritual context of human life; initiation science; the course of the year; and community building. As a foundation for an artistic school, he creates a series of pastel sketches. Lecture cycles: *The Anthroposophical Movement; Initiation Science* (CW 227) (in England at the Penmaenmawr Summer School); *The Four Seasons and the Archangels* (CW 229); *Harmony of the Creative Word* (CW 230); *The Supersensible Human* (CW 231), given in Holland for the founding of the Dutch society. On November 10, in response to the failed Hitler-Ludendorff putsch in Munich, Steiner closes his Berlin residence and moves the *Philosophisch-Anthroposophisch Verlag* (Press) to Dornach. On December 9, Steiner begins the serialization of his *Autobiography: The Course of My Life* (CW 28) in *Das Goetheanum*. It will continue to appear weekly, without a break, until his death. Late December–early January: Rudolf Steiner re-founds the Anthroposophical Society (about 12,000 members internationally) and takes over its leadership. The new board members are: Marie Steiner, Ita Wegman, Albert Steffen, Elizabeth Vreede, and Guenther Wachsmuth. (See *The Christmas Meeting for the Founding of the General Anthroposophical Society*, CW 260). Accompanying lectures: *Mystery Knowledge and Mystery Centers* (CW 232); *World History in the Light of Anthroposophy* (CW 233). December 25: the Foundation Stone is laid (in the hearts of members) in the form of the 'Foundation Stone Meditation.'

1924: January 1: having founded the Anthroposophical Society and taken over its leadership, Rudolf Steiner has the task of 'reforming' it. The process begins with a weekly newssheet ('What's Happening in the Anthroposophical Society') in which Rudolf Steiner's 'Letters to Members' and 'Anthroposophical Leading Thoughts' appear (CW 26). The next step is the creation of a new esoteric class, the 'first class' of the 'University of Spiritual Science' (which was to have been followed, had Rudolf Steiner lived longer, by two more advanced classes). Then comes a new language for Anthroposophy—practical, phenomenological, and direct; and Rudolf Steiner creates the model for the second Goetheanum. He begins the series of extensive 'karma' lectures (CW 235–40); and finally, responding to needs, he creates two new initiatives: biodynamic agriculture and curative education. After the middle of the year, rumors begin to circulate regarding Steiner's health. Lectures: January–February, *Anthroposophy* (CW 234); February: *Tone Eurythmy* (CW 278); June: *The Agriculture Course* (CW 327); June–July: *Speech Eurythmy* (CW 279); *Curative Education* (CW 317); August: (England, 'Second International Summer School'), *Initiation Consciousness: True and False Paths in Spiritual Investigation* (CW 243); September: *Pastoral Medicine* (CW 318). On September 26, for the first time, Rudolf Steiner cancels a lecture. On September 28, he gives his last lecture. On September 29, he withdraws to his studio in the carpenter's shop; now he is definitively ill. Cared for by Ita Wegman, he continues working, however, and writing the weekly installments of his *Autobiography* and *Letters to the Members/Leading Thoughts* (CW 26).

1925:   Rudolf Steiner, while continuing to work, continues to weaken. He finishes *Extending Practical Medicine* (CW 27) with Ita Wegman.

On March 30, around ten in the morning, Rudolf Steiner dies.

INDEX

PLATES

Plate 1

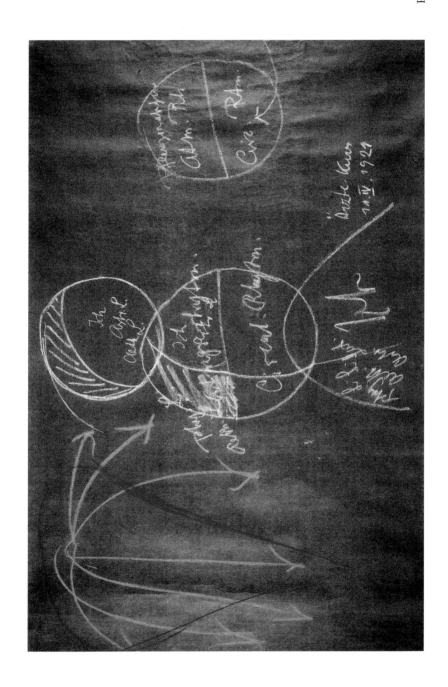

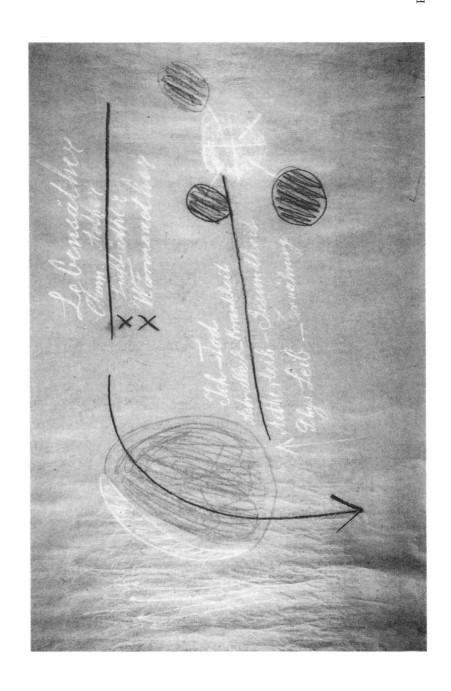

Plate 2

Plate 3

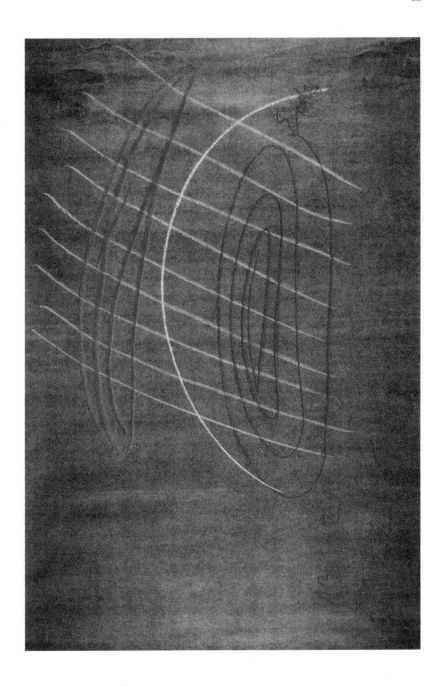

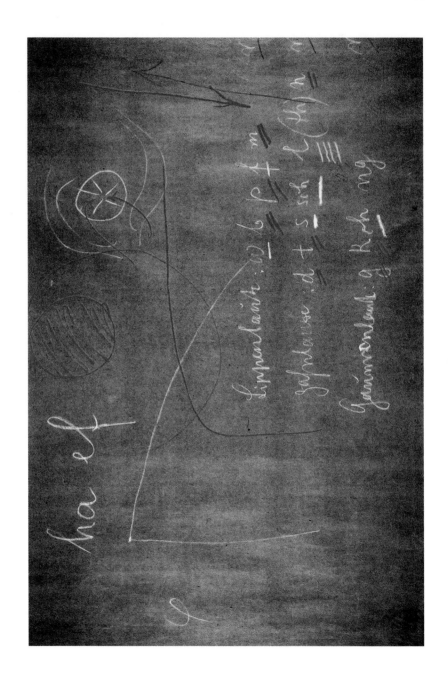

Plate 4

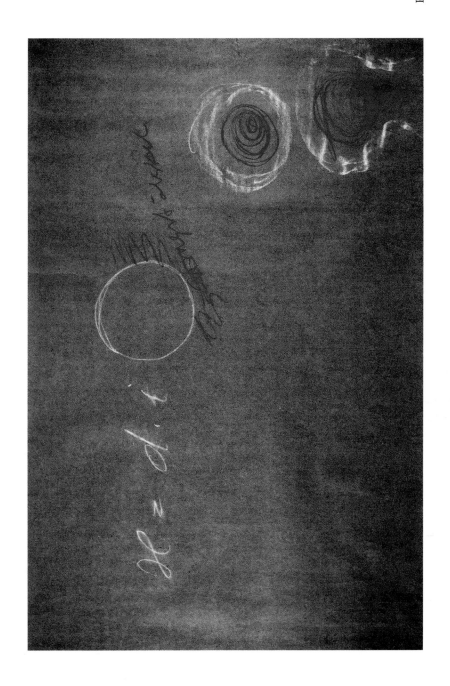

Plate 5

Plate 6

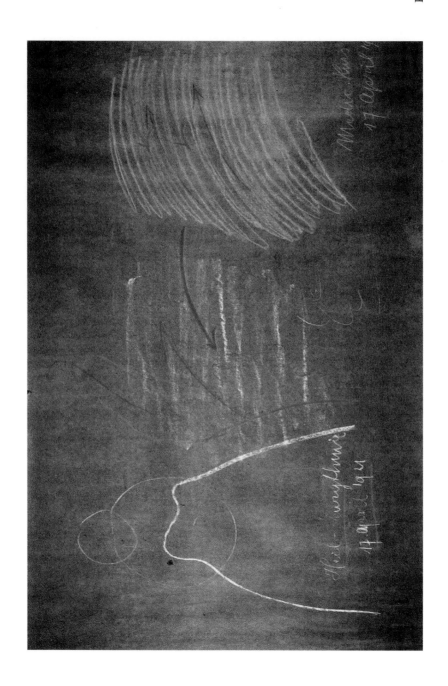

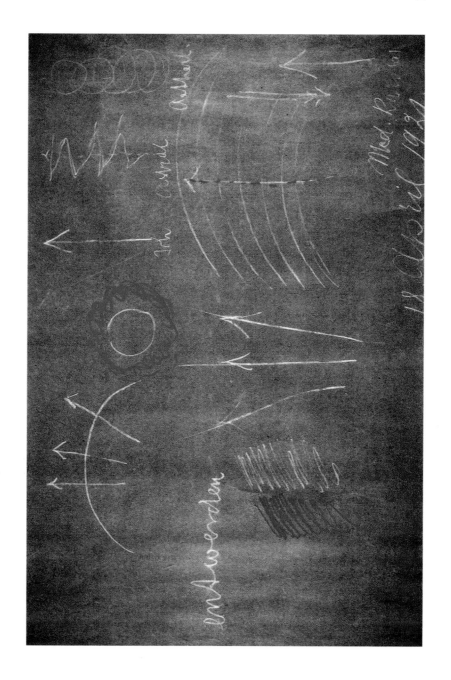

Plate 7